D1326316

An Atlas of Investigation and Management
ALLERGY

An Atlas of Investigation and Management

ALLERGY

S Hasan Arshad
North Staffordshire University Hospital
Stoke-on-Trent, Staffordshire, UK

Stephen T Holgate
Southampton General Hospital
Southampton, UK

N Franklin Adkinson, Jr
John Hopkins Asthma and Allergy Centre
Baltimore, MD, USA

K Suresh Babu
Southampton General Hospital
Southampton, UK

CLINICAL PUBLISHING

OXFORD

Distributed worldwide by
Taylor & Francis Ltd
Boca Raton   London   New York   Washington D.C.

Clinical Publishing
An imprint of Atlas Medical Publishing Ltd
Oxford Centre for Innovation
Mill Street, Oxford OX2 0JX, UK

Tel: +44 1865 811116
Fax: +44 1865 251550
Web: www.clinicalpublishing.co.uk

Distributed by:

Taylor & Francis Ltd
6000 Broken Sound Parkway NW, Suite 300
Boca Raton, FL 33487, USA
E-mail: orders@crcpress.com

Taylor & Francis Ltd
23–25 Blades Court
Deodar Road
London SW15 2NU, UK
E-mail: uk.tandf@thomsonpublishingservices.co.uk

A catalogue record for this book is available from the British Library

ISBN 1 904392 24 5

**The publisher makes no representation, express or implied, that the dosages
in this book are correct. Readers must therefore always check the product
information and clinical procedures with the most up-to-date published product
information and data sheets provided by the manufacturers and the most recent
codes of conduct and safety regulations. The authors and the publisher do not
accept any liability for any errors in the text or for the misuse or misapplication
of material in this work.**

Printed in Spain

Contents

Preface

The last 30 years have witnessed an unprecedented increase in the prevalence of all allergic disease that includes asthma, allergic rhinoconjunctivitis, drug and food allergy, anaphylaxis, occupational allergy, and allergic skin disease manifesting as atopic eczema and urticaria. While there is much debate about why this 'epidemic' has occurred, the highest prevalence and greatest change in demography appears to be linked to aspects of the Western lifestyle that not only includes altered exposure to micro-organisms, which is frequently cited as the cause for the changing trends, but also changes in housing, drug use, and diet, as well as indoor and outdoor air pollutants. It is most likely that more than one factor is involved in driving the trends.

Irrespective of the underlying cause(s), allergic disease has now assumed public health proportions affecting all age groups and often manifesting as multiple organ disease. Indeed, complex allergy often presents a diagnostic and therapeutic challenge. Since allergy has such protean manifestations it often falls not only within the domain of organ-based specialists, but also general practitioners, immunologists, and those specializing in allergy. All such professionals will find this Atlas an aid to the diagnosis and management of allergy.

With the aid of clear diagrams and ample clinical and pathological illustrations, this Atlas describes the mechanisms, epidemiology, diagnosis, and treatment of all of the common allergies. Great care has been taken to draw out the most salient features of each of the disorders and to present them in a way that will enhance learning and recall memory.

While there are many books on allergy, both small and large, this Atlas fills a unique niche in providing an accessible source of up-to-date information. This book is of special value to medical students and those in post-graduate training, as well as to practitioners who wish for an easy-to-use, illustrated reference source.

We are extremely grateful to our patients who co-operated in this effort and it is their interest that has made this unique book possible. We hope you find its content valuable. We are always pleased to receive comments, especially if you have any useful suggestions for future revisions.

SH Arshad
ST Holgate
NF Adkinson, Jr
KS Babu

Acknowledgements

The authors would like to express their gratitude to patients attending the David Hide Asthma and Allergy Centre for agreeing to have their photographs published in this Atlas.

The authors are also indebted to Mrs Sharon Matthews and the nursing staff of the Centre for their invaluable help in the collection of many of the photographs.

Abbreviations

ACD allergic contact dematitis
AD atopic dermatitis
ADR adverse drug reaction
AHR airway hyper-responsiveness
AIDS aquired immunodeficiency syndrome
ALL acute lymphoblastic leukaemia
APC antigen-presenting cell
ARDS adult respiratory distress syndrome
ARIA Allergic Rhinitis and its Impact on Asthma (Study)
BALF bronchoalveolar lavage fluid
BHR bronchial hyper-responsiveness
BPT bronchial provocation test
CD   contact dermatitis
CLA cutaneous lymphocyte-associated antigen
CLL chronic lymphocytic leukaemia
CS corticosteroids
DBPCFC double blind, placebo controlled food challenge
DH dermatitis herpetiformis
DNA deoxyribonucleic acid
DPI dry powder inhaler
ECP eosinophil cationic protein
ECRHS European Community Respiratory Health Survey
EDN eosinophil-derived neurotoxin
ELISA enzyme linked immunosorbent assay
EPO eosinophil peroxidase
FEV_1 forced expiratory volume in 1 second
FGF fibroblast growth factor
FVC forced vital capacity
GALT gut associated lymphoid tissue
GI gastrointestinal
GM-CSF granulocytic monocyte colony stimulating factor
HDM house dust mite
HIV human immunodeficiency virus
HLA human leucocyte antigen
H/O history of
HPA hypothalamopituitary axis
ICAM intercellular adhesion molecule

ID intradermal (test)
Ig immunoglobulin
IL interleukin
i.m. intramuscular
IMN infectious mononucleosis
INF interferon
ISAAC International Study of Asthma and Allergies in Childhood
i.v. intravenous
LABA long-acting beta agonist
LT leukotriene
MBP major basic protein
MCP monocyte chemotactic protein
MCT mast cell tryptase
MCTC mast cell tryptase, chymase
MDI metered-dose inhaler
MHC major histocompatibility complex
MIP 1α macrophage inflammatory protein 1 alpha
NARES non-allergic rhinitis with eosinophilic syndrome
NK natural killer (-cell)
NO nitric oxide
(i)NOS (inducible) nitric oxide synthase
NSAID non-steroidal anti-inflammatory drug
OCP oral contraceptive pill
PAF platelet activating factor
PAR perennial allergic rhinitis
PC_{20} provocation concentration (20% decrease in FEV_1)
PD_{20} provocation dose (20% decrease in FEV_1)
PDE phosphodiesterase
PEF peak expiratory flow
PEFR peak expiratory flow rate
PG prostaglandin
PRIST paper radioimmunosorbent assay
RIA radioimmunoassay
RAST radio allergen sorbent test
SALT skin associated lymphoid tissue
SAR seasonal allergic rhinitis

s.c. subcutaneous
SCF stem cell factor
SIT specific injection immunotherapy
SJS Steven–Johnson syndrome
SPT skin prick test
sRaw specific airway resistance
TCR T-cell receptor

TEN toxic epidermal necrolysis
TGF-β tissue growth factor-beta
THO T-helper (cells)
TNF-α tumour necrosis factor-alpha
VCAM vascular cell adhesion molecule
VLA very late antigen

Chapter 1

Introduction

An allergy is an immunologically-mediated adverse reaction to a foreign substance, usually a protein. Allergic reactions can affect almost any tissue or organ in the body, with clinical manifestations depending on the target organ. For example, asthma is the result of an allergic reaction affecting lower airways. When the nose and eyes are targeted, it manifests clinically as allergic rhinoconjunctivitis. Skin manifestations include: allergic maculopapular rash, urticaria, and angioedema. Systemic reactions may result in anaphylaxis.

Clinical manifestations of allergic diseases

Common clinical manifestations of allergy include asthma, atopic dermatitis, allergic rhinitis, and urticaria/angioedema.

Asthma

Experts from the National Institutes of Health defined asthma as:

'... a chronic inflammatory disorder of the airways in which many cells and cellular elements play a role, in particular, mast cells, eosinophils, T lymphocytes, macrophages, neutrophils, and epithelial cells. In susceptible individuals, this inflammation causes recurrent episodes of wheezing, breathlessness, chest tightness, and coughing, particularly at night or in the early morning. These episodes are usually associated with widespread but variable airway obstruction that is often reversible either spontaneously or with treatment. The inflammation also causes an associated increase in the existing bronchial hyper-responsiveness to a variety of stimuli.' (National Institutes of Health [1997] *Guidelines for the Diagnosis and Management of Asthma*. NIH Publication 97-4051A, Bethesda, Maryland.)

In severe asthma, airway obstruction can be extreme with occasionally fatal outcome (**1.1**). Airway obstruction in asthma has three major components: hypertrophy and contraction of the bronchial smooth muscle, mucosal oedema, and mucous plugging.

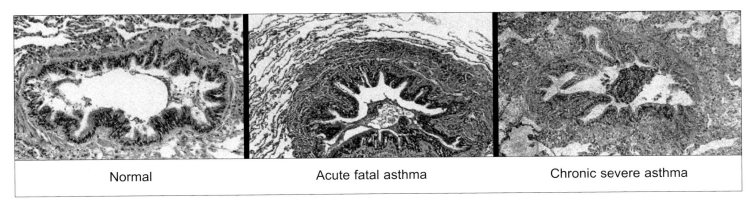

| Normal | Acute fatal asthma | Chronic severe asthma |

1.1 Airway in a normal subject and in those with severe asthma.

Definition of atopy and sensitization

Atopy is the genetic predisposition to produce Immunoglobulin E (IgE) antibodies on exposure to allergens.

Sensitization is the state where, following exposure to the allergens, the immune system is primed to produce IgE antibodies specific to that allergen.

Atopic dermatitis

Atopic dermatitis (AD) or atopic eczema is a chronic relapsing inflammatory skin condition with pruritis, and with typical morphology (erythematous vesicular lesions) and distribution (flexural areas, trunk) (**1.2**). However, both morphology and distribution can vary depending on the severity and duration of the disease, and age of the patient. It is often, but not always, associated with atopy.

Allergic rhinitis

Rhinitis is defined as inflammation of the nasal mucosa. It is characterized by nasal congestion, rhinorrhoea, sneezing, itching of the nose, and/or post-nasal drainage. It may be associated with ocular symptoms such as watering, congestion, and redness (rhinoconjunctivitis). Rhinitis may be allergic or non-allergic. Allergic rhinitis is diagnosed when symptoms are triggered by a recognized allergen. Nasal polyposis is a common complication of allergic rhinitis (**1.3**).

Urticaria and angioedema

Urticaria is an erythematous, palpable, itchy rash with distinct margins that may be localized to one area of the skin or generalized (**1.4**). The rash varies in shape and size, and may involve any area of the skin. Angioedema is subcutaneous or submucous oedema without distinct margins. It may occur with urticaria or as an isolated phenomenon. Typical episodes are of sudden onset, often itchy, and resolve to leave normal looking skin. Repeated episodes may occur (intermittent urticaria/angioedema) and if these continue beyond 6 weeks, it is termed chronic recurrent urticaria/angioedema.

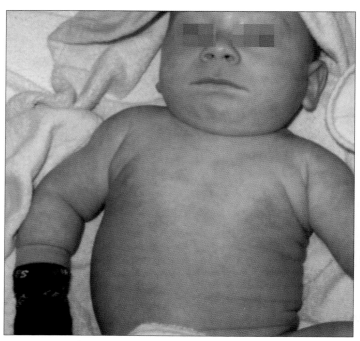

1.2 A patient with moderately severe atopic dermatitis.

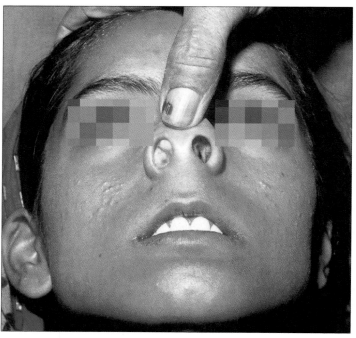

1.3 Right ethmoidal polyp due to allergic rhinitis. (Courtesy of Dr SH Abid.)

Prevalence of allergy

Allergic diseases are extremely common with nearly 50% of the population being affected at some time during their life. In several studies, the prevalence of sensitization to common allergens has been shown to be 20–40%.

Food allergy and atopic eczema is common in early childhood. These atopic children are at a higher risk of developing asthma and rhinitis in later childhood and early adult life. Allergic manifestations can be life-threatening such as severe asthma and anaphylactic reactions.

Asthma affects 10–15% of children and 5–10% of adults

(1.3 million children and 1.8 million adults in the UK are affected). Allergic rhinitis is observed in 10–20% of unselected population and atopic eczema in 5–10%, depending on the age and population studied. Perceived food allergy is extremely common and reported by 20–25% of the population. However, this is confirmed by double blind food challenges in only 2–7%. The true prevalence depends on the age and it is more common in young children.

Figures **1.5** and **1.6** show data from longitudinal follow-up studies of a whole population birth cohort. Children were

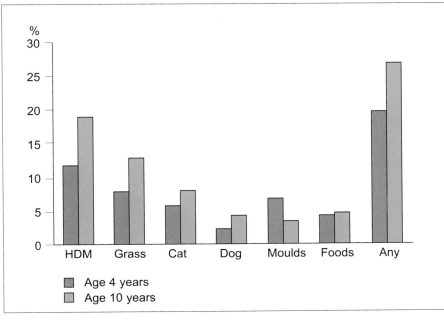

1.4 A patient with generalized urticaria.

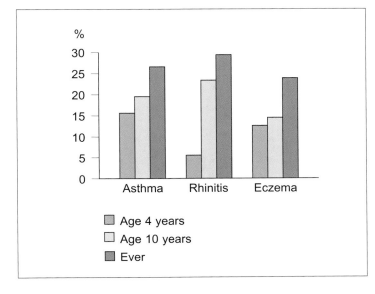

1.5 Period (age 4 and 10 years) and cumulative (ever) prevalence of allergic symptoms. (Data from the Isle of Wight whole population birth cohort.)

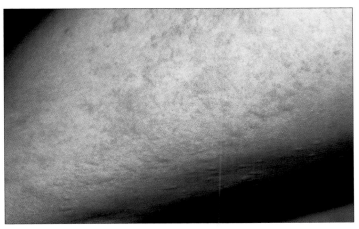

1.6 Sensitization to common allergens at ages 4 and 10 years in an unselected population. (HDM, house dust mite.) (Data from the Isle of Wight birth cohort.)

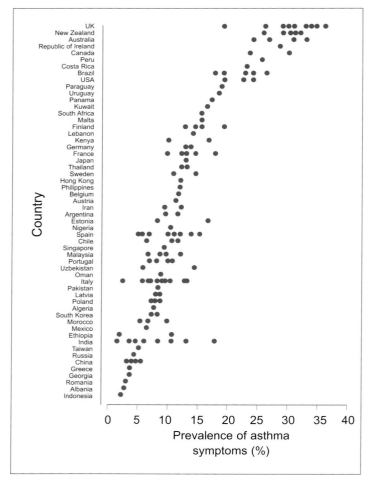

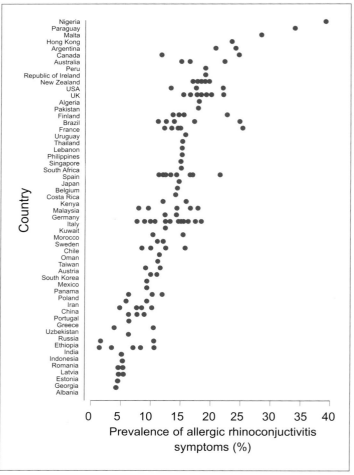

1.7 Twelve-month prevalences of self-reported asthma symptoms from written questionnaires. (Data derived from Beasley *et al.* [1998]. Worldwide variation in prevalence of symptoms of asthma, allergic rhinoconjunctivitis, and atopic eczema: ISAAC. *The Lancet,* **351(9111)**:1225–33.)

1.8 Twelve-month prevalences of allergic rhinoconjuctivitis symptoms. (Data derived from Beasley *et al.* [1998]. Worldwide variation in prevalence of symptoms of asthma, allergic rhinoconjunctivitis, and atopic eczema: ISAAC. *The Lancet,* **351(9111)**:1225–33.)

seen at regular intervals from birth to 10 years of age, thus reducing selection and re-call bias. They were also skin prick tested for 14 common food and inhalant allergens at 4 and 10 years of age. This prospective study confirmed a higher lifetime prevalence of allergic diseases during the first decade of life. Sensitization to at least one allergen was 20% at 4 years and increased to nearly 30% at 10 years of age.

World wide prevalence

As noted above, the prevalence of asthma and allergy showed wide variations in different populations, but these studies were not directly comparable, as study tools were often neither standardized nor validated. The inception of ISAAC (International Study of Asthma and Allergies in Childhood) using standardized questionnaire material has helped to reduce this problem. During the 1990s, the prevalence of asthma, atopic dermatitis, and rhinitis was

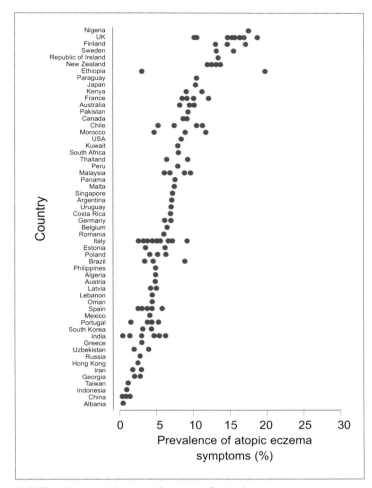

1.9 Twelve-month prevalences of atopic eczema symptoms. (Data derived from Beasley *et al*. [1998]. Worldwide variation in prevalence of symptoms of asthma, allergic rhinoconjunctivitis, and atopic eczema: ISAAC. *The Lancet,* **351(9111)**:1225–33.)

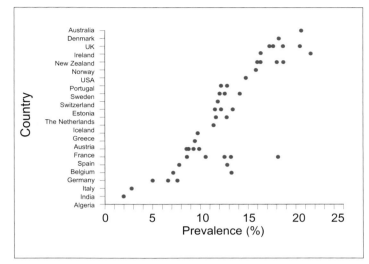

1.10 Prevalence of asthma in adults. In adults, as in children, asthma prevalence varied widely with Australia, Denmark, and UK showing highest prevalences, whereas developing countries such as India and Algeria showed lowest prevalence of asthma. Unfortunately, only a few countries outside Europe and Australia/New Zealand were included in the original study. However, several reports from countries around the world have since been published, using the European Community Respiratory Health Survey questionnaire, confirming differing prevalence across the globe. (Data derived from European Community Respiratory Health Survey [1996], *Eur Respir J,* **9**:687–95.)

assessed in several countries.

Figures **1.7**–**1.9** show data from the ISAAC study. The great advantage of the ISAAC study is its true international nature, with the same study tools being used throughout the world. Thus, reliable information is obtained on allergy related symptoms and diseases such as wheezing, asthma, atopic eczema, and allergic rhinoconjunctivitis. Importantly, data from different countries and populations could be compared with a degree of confidence. This study confirmed a wide variation in prevalence of all allergic manifestations. For example, asthma prevalence varied from <5% (Indonesia and Albania) to >35% (UK).

These studies were carried out in children. In adults, the European Community Respiratory Health Survey, using standardized questionnaires, assessed and compared the prevalence of asthma in several countries (**1.10**).

Rise in prevalence

Studies have consistently shown an increasing prevalence of allergic disease in recent decades. This is independent of the increasing awareness of allergy (and thus increase in reported symptoms) and changes in diagnostic criteria. Although there is considerable variation in the prevalence between countries (presumably due to different diagnostic criteria), the two observations in the same population used similar methodologies and yet showed a consistent pattern of rise in prevalence (**1.11**).

Recent reports, however, indicate that the prevalence may have reached a peak; the last few years have shown a slight decline in prevalence in some developed countries. Figure **1.12** shows data from a recent Canadian study. Asthma prevalence was highest in the pre-school age children, and continued to show a slight increase in prevalence over the study period. However, in other age groups there seems to be a trend of increased prevalence from 1991–1995 and

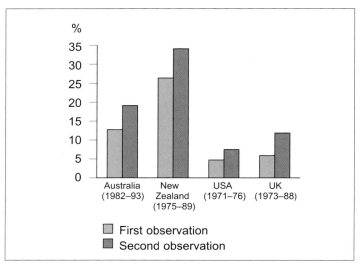

1.11 Increase in the prevalence of diagnosed asthma in developed countries. These studies were done in the same population using identical methodologies.

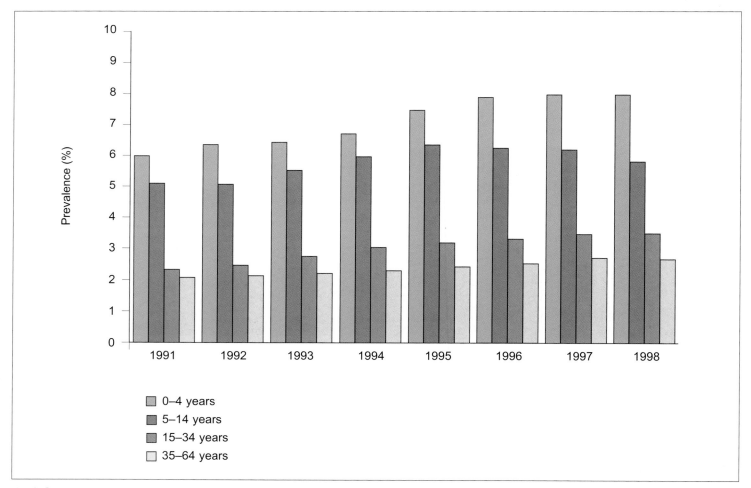

1.12 Stabilization of an increasing trend in physician-diagnosed asthma prevalence in Saskatchewan, Canada, 1991–98. (Data derived from Senthilselvan A, *et al.* [2003]. Stabilization of an increasing trend in physician-diagnosed asthma prevalence in Saskatchewan, 1991 to 1998. *Chest*, **124(2)**:438–48.)

then stabilization between 1995–1998. It may be too early to say if the rise in asthma prevalence, observed consistently during the 1960s through the early 1990s, has reached a plateau.

Expression of allergic diseases

Development of an allergy depends on genetic and environmental factors. Genetic susceptibility is a prerequisite for the development of asthma and other allergic disorders, but the precise nature and location of these genes is still not fully understood. Allergic disorders are polygenetic diseases, and a large number of genes on several different chromosomes have been implicated. They may share genes which regulate atopic immune responses, such as those for interleukin (IL)-4, IL-13 and interferon gamma (INF-γ). Other relevant genes may be related to the target organ's structure or function. For example, for asthma these may determine airway responsiveness or regulate airway epithelial and mesenchymal function. A certain combination or series of combinations of genes or genetic polymorphisms may be required for the phenotypic expression.

Simply having the right combination of genes is not enough, however. A number of environmental exposures, especially early in life, are known to promote or protect the development of allergy and asthma. It is highly likely that an interaction of genetic and environmental factors determines the eventual phenotypic outcome in terms of the type and number of allergic manifestations, and may also influence the degree of severity and prognosis (**1.13**).

Initial allergen exposure causes sensitization in individuals who are genetically predisposed. Atopy or sensitization to allergens is common and may occur in 40–50% of the general population. Those with genetic predisposition to a particular target organ disease, such as asthma or rhinitis, develop a specific clinical disease. Exposure to certain environmental factors may promote or protect against this development. Further exposure to allergens or pollutant may result in symptoms or exacerbation. (**1.14**).

It is important to note that the degree of allergen exposure required to cause sensitization is not known, and may vary from allergen to allergen. In some cases, a higher exposure may indeed be protective by stimulating immune tolerance mechanisms. Recent studies suggest that a higher exposure to the cat allergen may protect against the development of sensitization. However, the same cannot be said about other common allergens, such as pollens, house dust mites, or cockroaches.

Atopy, as defined by positive skin prick test or presence of specific IgE to common allergens, is an important risk factor for the development of asthma and allergic disease (**1.15, 1.16**). However, atopy can be present without clinical manifestation (asymptomatic sensitization). These asymptomatically sensitized children, when followed over a period of several years, show a high rate of development of clinical disease. It is not known why some of these children develop clinical manifestations, whereas others remain asymptomatic.

1.13 Genetic and environmental risk factors for the development of asthma. (BHR, bronchial hyper-responsiveness.)

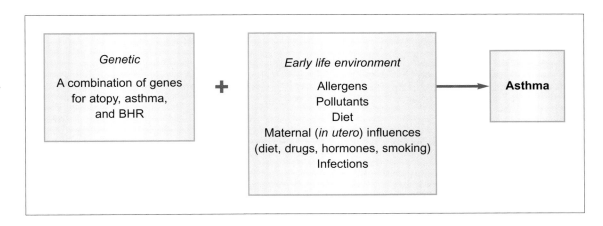

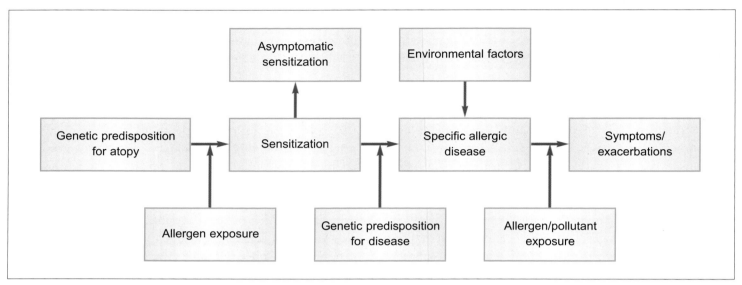

1.14 Development of sensitization and clinical allergic disease.

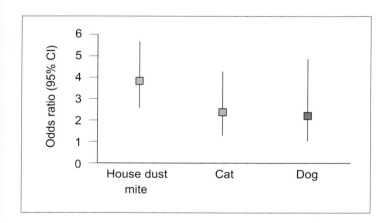

1.15 The risk of asthma (odds ratios and their 95% confidence intervals) in 10-year-old children sensitized (on skin prick test) to three common allergens: house dust mites, cats, and dogs.

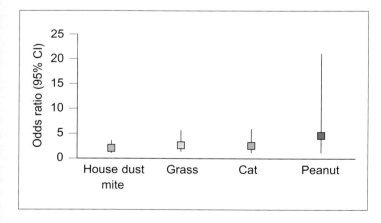

1.16 The risk of atopic dermatitis (odds ratios and their 95% confidence intervals) in 4-year-old children sensitized (on skin prick test) to four common allergens: house dust mites, grasses, cats, and peanuts.

Allergic immune responses

Pluripotent stem cells in the bone marrow give rise to all lineages of immune cells (**1.17**). The pluripotent stem cells give rise to lymphoid progenitors and the haematopoetic progenitors. While the haematopoetic progenitors are capable of maturing into granulocytes, erythrocytes, megakaryocytes and monocyte-dendritic series, the lymphoid progenitors mature into T-cells, B-cells and natural killer- (NK-) cells. The T-cell progenitors leave the bone marrow and home into the thymus to develop into αβ T-cells and γδ T-cells.

Regulation of stem cell differentiation occurs through interaction with various cell surface receptors and cytokines. Cytokines have pleiotropic effects on the haematopoetic and lymphoid cell development, affecting both the growth and maintenance of the pluripotent stem cells, as well as the differentiation of specific lineages.

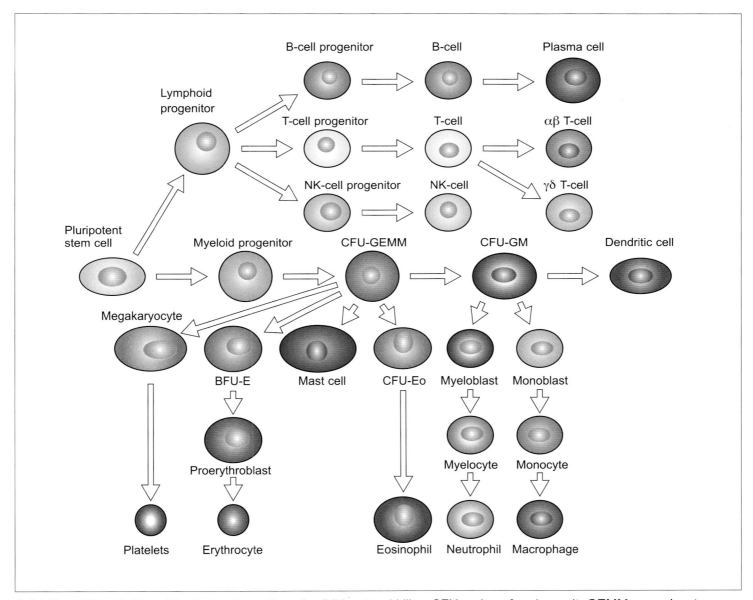

1.17 The differentiation of the haematopoetic cells. (NK, natural killer; CFU, colony forming unit; GEMM, granulocyte, erythroid, monocytic–dendritic, and megakaryocytic lineage; BFU-E, blast forming unit erythroid; Eo, eosinophil.)

Antigen-presenting cells

Cells that act as antigen-presenting cells (APCs) include a diverse group of leucocytes, such as monocytes, macrophages, dendritic cells, and B-cells (**1.18**). In addition, endothelial and epithelial cells can acquire antigen presenting abilities. APCs are found predominantly in the lymphoid organs and in the skin. Dendritic cells reside as immature cells in the skin, intestinal mucosa, lungs, and the genitourinary tract.

The three types of APCs present different sets of antigens and also serve to activate T-cells at different points during the immune response. Most (including B-cells, macrophages, and dendritic cells), express major histocompatibility complex (MHC) class II antigens on their surface. These are important for communication with T-cells and subsequent T-cell activation. Although many cells do not normally express MHC class II antigens, certain cytokines can induce their expression and thereby potentiate antigen presentation. In addition to antigen presentation, the APCs provide co-stimulatory signals via B7.1 and B7.2.

Cells of the monocyte–macrophage system exist in the blood. Macrophages are more differentiated monocytes that are resident in the tissues. These cells express MHC class II molecules on their surface. They have phagocytic and cytotoxic functions. The microscopic shape of the macrophages depends upon their function. They have a flexible cytoskeleton that makes them ovoid during transit, and stellate, with engulfing surface projections, during phagocytosis.

B-cells are produced in the bone marrow and are distributed through the body in the lymph nodes. B-cells respond to the 'foreign' antigens of a pathogen by producing specific antibodies. B-cell receptors bind soluble antigens. The bound antigen molecules are engulfed into the B-cell by receptor-mediated endocytosis. The antigen is then digested into fragments which are displayed at the cell surface, nestled inside a class II histocompatibility molecule. Helper T-cells, specific to this structure, bind the B-cell and secrete lymphokines.

Eosinophils and mast cells

Eosinophils (**1.19**) comprise 2–5% of white cells. Their peak production occurs at night. The mean generation time for eosinophils in the bone marrow is approximately 2–6 days. The cytokines important in the development of eosinophils include granulocyte monocyte colony stimulating factor (GM-CSF), IL-3, and IL-5. While GM-CSF and IL-3 promote eosinophil differentiation and growth, IL-5 has lineage-specific effects. The eosinophil cytoplasm contains large ellipsoid granules with an electron-dense crystalline nucleus and partially permeable matrix. In addition to these large primary crystalloid granules, there is another granule type that is smaller and lacks the crystalline nucleus. The large specific granules contain four dominant proteins: major basic protein (MBP), eosinophil cationic protein (ECP), eosinophil-derived neurotoxin (EDN), and eosinophil peroxidase (EPO). In addition, the specific granules contain preformed stores of cytokines and chemokines, histaminase, and lysozomal enzymes. The adhesion of eosinophils to endothelium include CD18-dependent pathways, interaction between E-selectin and P-selectin, and adherence to vascular cell adhesion molecule

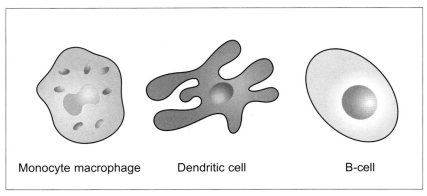

| Monocyte macrophage | Dendritic cell | B-cell |

1.18 Antigen-presenting cells involved in allergic immune response.

(VCAM) by means of very late antigen 4 (VLA-4) expressed on the eosinophil. Eosinophils contribute to immune responses to parasitic infections and contribute to inflammation in allergic diseases.

The pro-inflammatory effector function of eosinophils has been supported by an extensive number of studies. One of the important observations is that the treatment of monkeys with an anti-ICAM-1 monoclonal antibody clearly inhibited allergen-induced lung eosinophil influx and also prevented airway hyper-responsiveness. Similar findings were obtained following treatment with an anti-IL-5 antibody (TRFK-5), reinforcing the interpretation that there is indeed a causal link between eosinophilia and airway hyper-reactivity. However, there is evidence opposing this concept. It has been determined that blocking the effects of IL-5 by an anti-IL-5 antibody, mepolizumab, or a soluble IL-5 receptor, suppresses allergen-induced bronchoalveolar lavage fluid (BALF) eosinophilia with little effect on bronchial hyper-reactivity. This puts into question the functional role of eosinophils in allergic diseases.

Mast cells (**1.19**) are found only in tissues and they contain abundant granules. The stem cell factor is essential for mast cell development and survival, and influences mast cell function. Mast cells are 6–12 μm in diameter and the cytoplasm contains granules and crystals alone, or in combination. The surface of mast cells have receptors for IgE, cytokines, growth factors, and cell adhesion structures. There are two different types of mast cells which are designated mucosal or connective tissue, based on their location. Mast cells contain granules which store mediators of inflammation. Degranulation of mast cells can be induced by physical trauma, temperature, toxins, proteases, and immune-mediated mechanisms involving the aggregation of IgE bound to high-affinity receptors (FcεRI) on the surface of these cells. The effects of degranulation by cross-linking of cell surface IgE by antigens releases heparin, histamine, and other mediators to initiate an immediate allergic response. Upon stimulation, mast cells release cytokines, including tumour necrosis factor-alpha (TNF-α) and IL-4, that can modulate adhesion molecules on endothelial cells.

Mast cells originate from CD34+ progenitor cells in the bone marrow. Mast cells are widely distributed throughout the body in both connective tissue and at mucosal surfaces. The predominant mast cell subtype in the lung contains tryptase (MCT), although tryptase and chymase mast cells (MCTC) are also present. Mast cell activation occurs when IgE, bound to the high-affinity IgE Fc receptor (FcεRI) on mast cells, is cross-linked by allergens triggering mast cell degranulation. This results in the release of preformed granule-derived mediators and neutral proteases, the synthesis and release of newly formed lipid products, and the transcription of numerous cytokines (*Table 1.1*, p13). In addition to this conventional IgE-dependent mast cell activation, recent studies indicate that allergens, such as Der p 1 (a serine protease), as well as neuropeptides, eosinophil products, defensins, and changes in osmolality can induce mast cell histamine and cytokine secretion directly through IgE-independent mechanisms. Antigen-specific mast cell activation results in an immediate response while the late-phase response is a consequence of cytokines and other mediators derived from these cells or other cells recruited to the site of inflammation (**1.20**).

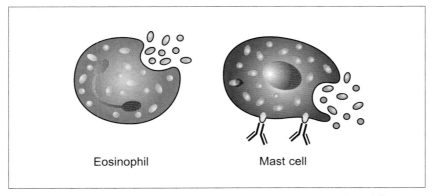

Eosinophil   Mast cell

1.19 Effector cells of the allergic immune responses: eosinophils and mast cells.

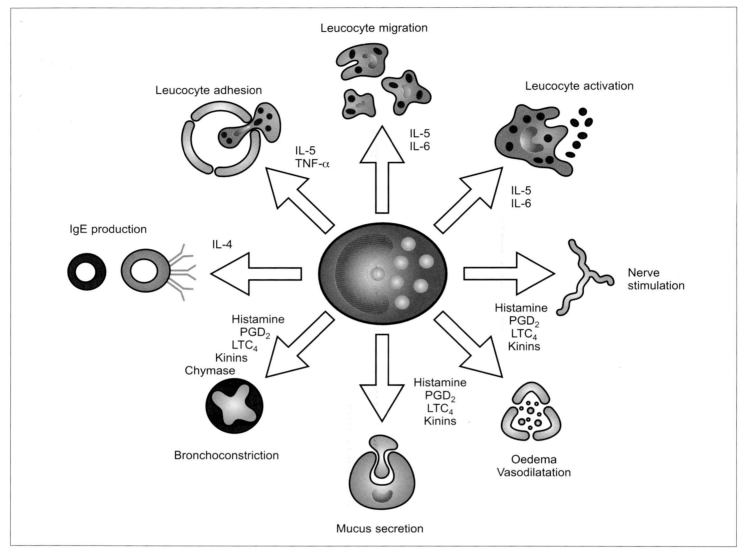

1.20 The effects of mast cell mediators. (Ig, immunoglobulin; IL, interleukin; LT, leukotriene; PG, prostaglandin; TNF-α, tumour necrosis factor-alpha.)

Lymphocytes

Lymphocytes are divided into T- and B-cells. In the early stages of development, T-cell precursors migrate to the thymus. T-cells are divided into subsets based on their surface expression of CD4 and CD8. CD4 T-cells recognize antigens in the context of MHC class II molecules and CD8 cells recognize antigens presented by class I molecules. T-cells express a clonal antigen-specific receptor. The T-cell receptor (TCR) is in fact very similar to immunoglobulin. It has two paired polypeptide chains both of which have constant and variable portions and both of which are composed of immunoglobulin-like domain. B-cells represent 5–10% of lymphocytes and their cytoplasm is characterized by scattered ribosomes and isolated rough endoplasmic reticula. Plasma cells are the mature form of B-lymphocytes that secrete antibodies.

A small fraction (~2%) of the lymphocytes circulating in the blood are neither T- nor B-cells. Most of these are called NK-cells because they are already specialized to kill certain types of target cells, especially host cells that have become infected with a virus or have become cancerous (**1.21**). They express CD16 and/or CD56 antigens. They are found in the liver, spleen, lungs, blood, and gastrointestinal (GI) tract. NK-cells are activated by IL-2, IL-12, IL-15, or IL-18.

Table 1.1 Mast cell mediators in allergic disease

Mediators	*Biological effects*
Histamine	Bronchoconstriction, tissue oedema, mucus secretion, fibroblast and endothelial proliferation
Heparin	Anticoagulant, storage matrix for mast cell mediators, fibroblast activation
Tryptase	Generates c3a and bradykinin, increases BHR, activates collagenase, fibroblast proliferation
Chymase	Mucus secretion, extracellular matrix degradation
PGD_2	Bronchoconstriction, tissue oedema, mucus secretion
LTC_4	Bronchoconstriction, tissue oedema, mucus secretion
TNF-α	Neutrophil chemotaxis, MHC class II expression, increased expression of adhesion molecules, mucus secretion, increases IL-8 and IL-6 synthesis in fibroblasts
IL-4, IL-13	B-cell proliferation, increase IgE synthesis, activation of eosinophils
IL-5, GM-CSF	Eosinophil recruitment, activation, and survival
IL-6	IgE synthesis, differentiation of T-cells, mucus secretion
IL-8	Neutrophil chemotaxis
IL-16	T-cell chemotaxis
SCF	Growth, differentiation, and survival of mast cells
Basic FGF	Angiogenesis, fibroblast proliferation
MCP-1	Monocyte and T-cell chemotaxis
MIP-1α	Macrophage differentiation, neutrophil chemotaxis

BHR, bronchial hyper-responsiveness; FGF, fibroblast growth factor; GM-CSF, granulocyte monocyte colony stimulating factor; Ig, immunoglobulin; IL, interleukin; LT, leukotriene; MCP, monocyte chemotactic protein; MHC, major histocompatibility complex; MIP, macrophage inflammatory protein; PG, prostaglandin; SCF, stem cell factor; TNF-α, tumour necrosis factor-alpha

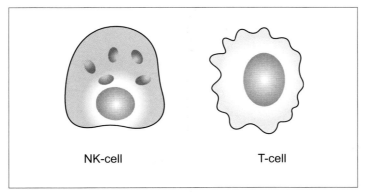

NK-cell   T-cell

1.21 Lymphocytes orchestrate the immune responses in both allergic and non-allergic inflammation.

Table 1.2 Characteristics of different classes of immunoglobulins

Property	IgM	IgG	IgA	IgE	IgD
Serum composition (%)	10	75	15	<0.01	<0.5
Structure	Pentamer	Monomer	Dimer	Monomer	Monomer
Complement fixation	+++	+	-	-	-
Opsoninization	+ (via complement)	+++	-	-	-
Allergic response	-	-	-	+	-
Mucosal secretion	-	-	+	-	-
Functions	Primary response Ig Fixes complement	Secondary response Ig Neutralizes toxins, virus Opsoninization	Secretory Ig Provides mucosal immunity	Immediate hypersensitivity Protection from helminthic infection	Uncertain
Increased in	Waldenstrom's macroglobinaemia Trypnosomiasis Actinomycosis Malaria IMN SLE Rheumatoid arthritis	Chronic granulomatous disease Infections Liver disease Malnutrition Dysproteinaemia Rheumatoid arthritis IgG myeloma	Wiskott–Aldrich syndrome Cirrhosis Chronic infections IgA myeloma	Eczema Hayfever Asthma Anaphylactic reaction IgE myeloma	Chronic infections
Decreased in	Agamma-globinaemia Lymphoproliferative disorders Dysgamma-globinaemia CLL IgG, IgA myeloma	Agamma-globinaemia Lymphoid aplasia Selective IgG, IgA deficiency Bence–Jones proteinaemia CLL	Heriditary telangiectasia Malabsorbtion syndromes ALL, CLL IgG myeloma	Congenital agamma-globinaemia	IgD myeloma

ALL, acute lymphoblastic leukaemia; CLL, chronic lymphocytic leukaemia; Ig, immunoglobulin; IMN, infectious mononucleosis; SLE, systemic lupus erythematosus

Immunoglobulins

Immunoglobulins are glycoprotein molecules which are produced by plasma cells and which function as antibodies. The immunoglobulins derive their name from the finding that when antibody-containing serum is placed in an electrical field, the antibodies responsible for immunity migrated with the globular proteins. All immunoglobulins have a four chain structure as their basic unit. They are composed of two identical light chains (23 kD) and two identical heavy chains (50–70 kD). The heavy and light chains can be divided into two regions based on variability in the amino acid sequences: the variable and the constant regions. Subtle structural differences in their antigen combining sites, or variable region, account for their unique antigen-binding specificities. There are five different classes of immunoglobulins (*Table 1.2*).

1.22 Interaction between an antigen-presenting cell and a lymphocyte.

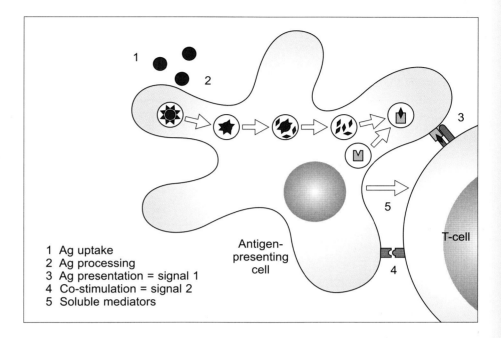

1 Ag uptake
2 Ag processing
3 Ag presentation = signal 1
4 Co-stimulation = signal 2
5 Soluble mediators

Antigen-presenting cell

T-cell

1.23 Class switching to IgE and B-cell proliferation.

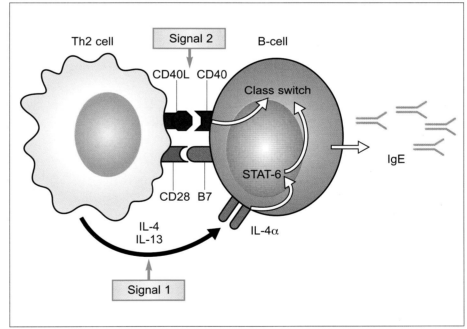

Antigen uptake

When a T- or B-cell engages an antigen through its antigen receptor an intra-cellular signal is generated (**1.22**). The first signal, which gives specificity to the immune response, is provided by the interaction of antigenic peptide–MHC complex with the TCR. The second antigen-independent co-stimulatory signal is delivered to T-cells by APCs to promote T-cell clonal expansion, cytokine secretion, and effector function. In the absence of the second signal,

antigen-specific lymphocytes fail to respond effectively, and are functionally inactivated and resistant to subsequent activation to the antigen.

Production of immunoglobulin E

IgE production requires at least two distinct signals (**1.23**). The first signal is provided by the cytokines IL-4 and IL-13. IL-4 is produced by T-cells, although mast cells, basophils, and eosinophils may also produce IL-4, whereas IL-13 is also produced by the NK-cells. IL-4 and IL-13 share the common α chain of the IL-4 receptor (IL-4α). Engagement of this moiety with either ligands results in translocation to the nucleus of the signal transducer and the activator of transcription 6 (STAT-6). These stimulate transcription of the Cε gene locus containing the exons encoding the constant region domains of the IgE ε heavy chain. The second signal is delivered by the interaction of CD40L on the surface of the T-cell with CD40, a co-stimulatory molecule on the B-cell membrane. This activates a genetic rearrangement (deletional switch recombination) that brings into proximity all the elements of a functional ε heavy chain. The product is a complete multi-exon gene encoding the full ε heavy chain. The combination of these signals causes class switching to IgE and B-cell proliferation.

Immunoglobulin E

IgE is the immunoglobulin involved in allergic reactions. IgE is commonly known as the 'reaginic' antibody. IgE is the least common immunoglobulin, since it binds very tightly to Fc receptors on basophils and mast cells, even before interacting with antigens and, secondly, due to the very small amount synthesized. Like other antibodies, IgE is comprised of two identical light chains and two identical heavy chains, each chain made up of 110 amino acids called immunoglobulin domains, covalently linked by disulphide

bonds (**1.24**). The L-chain has one N-terminal variable (VL) domain and one constant (CL) domain. Likewise, the H-chain consists of one N-terminal V (VH) domain and four C (CH) domains. The antibody class is determined by the CH sequence designated as Cε for IgE. A given B-cell produces an antibody with one specificity, as defined by the VL and VH combination, but during an antibody response, it can 'switch' classes. IgE has a profound effector function due to the fact that basophils and mast cells have high affinity receptors for the Fc portion of the molecule. IgE also binds to Fc receptors on the surface of eosinophils. This allows eosinophils to participate in antibody-dependent, cell-mediated cytotoxicity reactions against parasitic helminths.

IgE receptors and their interaction

Two classes of Fcε receptors have been identified, designated as FcεRI and FcεRII (or CD23) (**1.25**). The high-affinity receptors are predominantly expressed on mast cells, as well as basophils and APCs, and not on their precursors in circulation. The high affinity of these receptors (kD = 1–2 × 10^{-9} M) enables them to bind to IgE, despite its low serum concentrations. The FcεRI receptor has four polypeptide chains: an α-chain and a β-chain, and two identical disulfide-linked γ-chains. FcεRI interacts with the CH3/CH3 and CH4/CH4 domains of the IgE molecule via the two immunoglobulin-like domains of the a chain. FcεRI

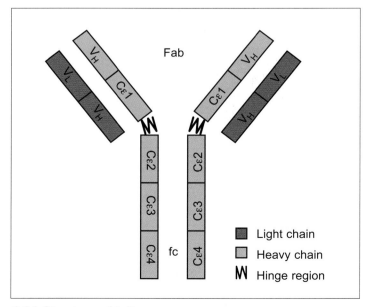

1.24 Structure of IgE.

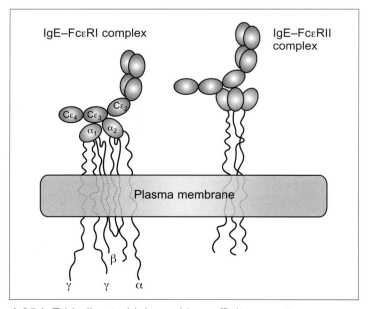

1.25 IgE binding to high- and low-affinity receptors.

either wraps around a single Cε3 domain to make contact with both sides, or it interacts with opposite faces of the Cε3 domains on one side of IgE. The β-chain spans the plasma membrane four times and the two γ-chains extend a considerable distance into the cytoplasm. Allergen-mediated cross-linkage of the bound IgE results in aggregation of the FcεRI receptors and rapid tyrosine phosphorylation, which initiates the process of mast cell degranulation.

FcεRII is the low-affinity IgE receptor with a kD of 1×10^{-6} M and is specific for the CH3/CH3 domain of the IgE. It belongs to the family of C-type lectins. CD23 is a 45-kD polypeptide chain with extracellular structural motifs, a transmembrane sequence, and a cytoplasmic tail. The cytoplasmic tail can be either of two types: CD23a and CD23b. Allergen cross-linkage of IgE bound to the FcεRII receptors results in activation of B-cells, eosinophils, and alveolar macrophages. Blockage of this receptor with a monoclonal antibody leads to diminished IgE secretion by the B-cells. Interestingly, CD23 appears to act both in the up-regulation and down-regulation of IgE synthesis, and atopic individuals have higher levels of CD23 on their lymphocytes and macrophages. CD23–IgE interaction provides an important mechanism whereby allergen-specific IgE can augment cellular and humoral immune responses in settings of recurrent allergen exposure.

Summary

When an antigen enters the body through the mucosal surfaces or skin, the antigen-presenting cells, such as macrophages, engulf the antigens. Cross linking of Fab fragments of two adjacent IgE antibodies, on the surface of the mast cells by the allergen, results in the degranulation and release of preformed (histamine, heparin) and newly synthesized mediators (prostaglandins, leukotrienes, platelet-activating factor, and bradykinin). The dose and route of allergen administration determine the type of IgE-mediated reaction. An allergen in the blood stream activates connective tissue mast cells throughout the body, leading to systemic release of histamine and other mediators which, in turn, leads to anaphylaxis (1.26). Subcutaneous administration causes a local inflammatory reaction. Inhaled allergens activate mucosal mast cells leading to broncho-constriction and increased mucous secretion. Ingested allergens lead to food allergy.

1.26 Type of allergic reaction/disease may depend on the characteristics of allergen and the route of administration.

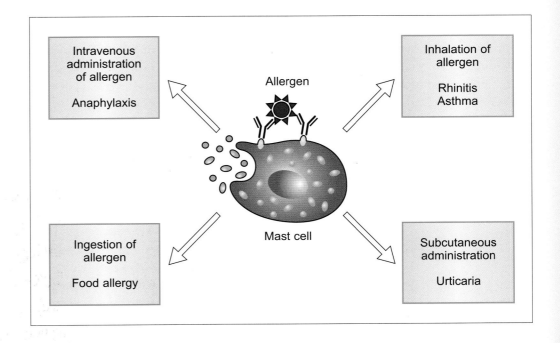

Allergens

A number of allergens are present in the air (aeroallergens) and, partly depending on the size of the particle, may cause upper or lower airway allergies. Systemic reactions to aeroallergens are rare. Allergens from food sources tend to cause GI or skin manifestations but, depending on the nature of the food allergen and sensitivity of the subject, may result in a systemic reaction. Allergens injected into the body, such as insect venom or drugs, often result in a systemic reaction. Allergens coming in contact with the skin may cause urticaria or contact dermatitis. However, there is considerable overlap and aeroallergens, such as house dust mites, may exacerbate atopic dermatitis in a sensitized individual, and food allergens may rarely cause asthma.

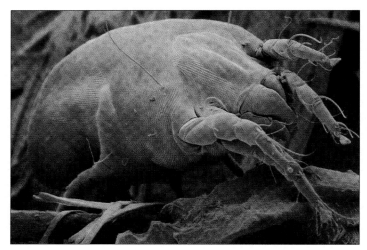

1.27 An electron microscopic photograph of a common house dust mite, *Dermatophagoides pteronyssinus*.

Aeroallergens

The most frequently encountered aeroallergens are: house dust mites, pollens (trees, grasses, and weeds), mould spores, and allergens of animal origin.

House dust mites

House dust mites are one of the most common allergens worldwide. These are eight legged, sightless creatures living in dust that accumulates in carpets, bedding, fabrics, mattresses, blankets, and pillows, as well as furniture and soft toys. House dust provides them with a habitat and contains their food source in the form of sloughed human skin. They are approximately 0.3 mm in length and are visible only by microscopic examination of the dust (**1.27**). Humidity and temperature are the most critical factors in the survival of the house dust mite population. There are two groups of important allergens derived from the common species of house dust mites: Group 1 (Der p 1 and Der f 1) and Group 2 (Der p 2 and Der f 2), isolated from *Dermatophagoides pteronyssinus* and *Der. farinae,* respectively. It is estimated that 20–30% of the European population is sensitized to *Der. pteronyssinus*. The presence of house dust mite sensitization is strongly associated with asthma and perennial allergic rhinitis. The role of house dust mites in atopic dermatitis remains unclear.

Pollen

Grass, tree, and weed pollens are some of the most common aeroallergens. Several species of grass, tree, and weed pollens have been identified as important in causing seasonal allergic rhinoconjunctivitis and pollen-induced asthma (**1.28**). A number of allergenic proteins have been identified as causing immune responses. Pollen allergens are water-soluble proteins or glycoproteins with a molecular weight of 10–70 kD. Most grass, tree, and weed species are wind-pollinated and release pollen grains over a short period of time. The airway exposure is highest during the peak flowering season, which is early to mid summer. Grass, tree, and weed pollen allergy may affect nearly 20% of the population.

1.28 (Right) Common species of pollen-bearing plants: **A** timothy grass (*Phleum pratense*); **B** rye grass (*Lolium perenne*); **C** meadow fescue (*Festuca pratensis*); **D** olive (*Olea europaea*); **E** grey alder (*Alnus incana*); **F** silver birch (*Betula pendula*); **G** hazel (*Corylus avellana*); **H** common stinging nettle (*Urtica dioica*); **I** common ragweed (*Ambrosia artemisiifolia*).

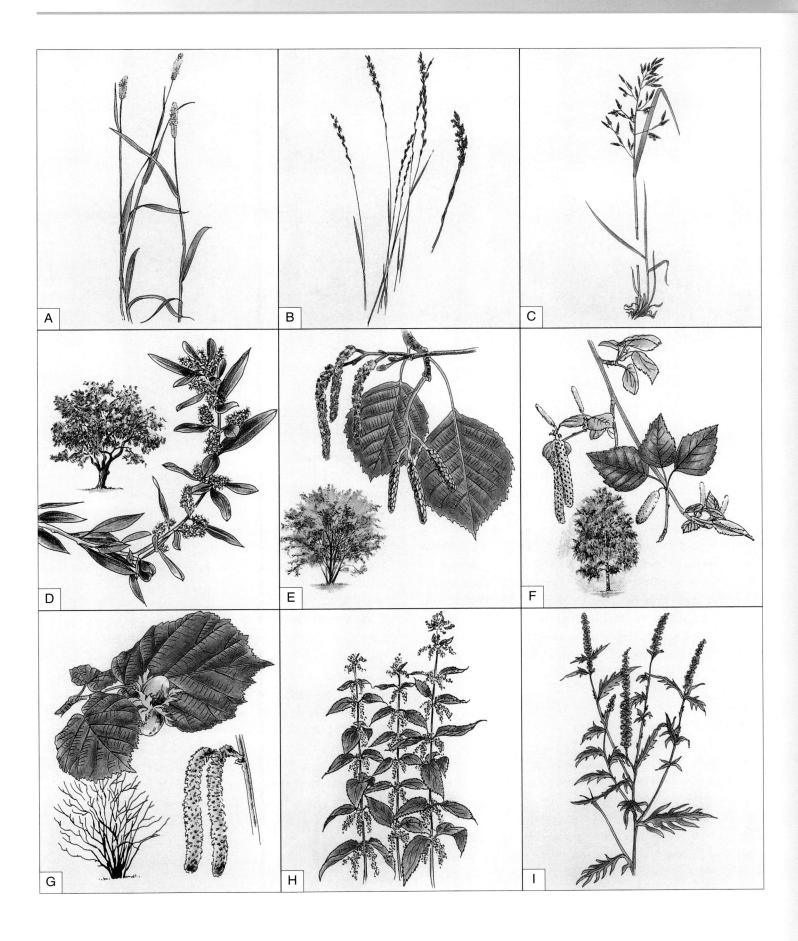

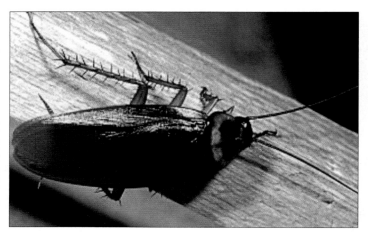

1.29 American cockroach, *Periplaneta americana.* (Courtesy of H Robertson, Iziko Museum of Cape Town, South Africa.)

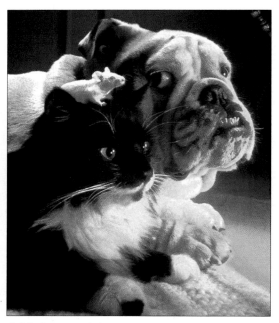

1.30 Cats and dogs are the most common furry pets responsible for allergy to animals.

Cockroach

Cockroaches are widely present in urban or inner-city areas and cockroach proteins are an important indoor allergen in these places. Two species of cockroaches, the American (*Periplaneta americana*) (**1.29**) and German (*Blattella germanica*) commonly inhabit the home and have a potential to cause sensitization. Important cockroach allergens are Bla g 1, with a molecular weight of 30 kD, and Bla g 2, with a molecular weight of 36 kD. Cockroach allergens can be detected anywhere in the house, but highest levels are usually found in kitchens and bathrooms. Sensitization to cockroach allergen has been shown to be an important risk factor for the development of asthma among inner-city residents.

Animal

In the Western world, nearly 50% of homes have cats and/or dogs as pets (**1.30**). These animals significantly contribute to indoor allergens. They produce allergenic proteins as secretions, excretions, or dander. Fel d 1 (a major cat allergen) and Can f 1 (a major dog allergen) can be easily measured in dust samples. Allergens can also accumulate from the urine of rodents (wild, domesticated, or laboratory). Sensitization to cat, dog, or mouse allergens is consistently associated with asthma.

Food allergens

Food allergens are almost always proteins. Potentially, any food can provoke a reaction. However, some foods are more allergenic than others, and these are responsible for most of the food allergic reactions. Common allergenic foods include: milk, egg, wheat, fish, and shellfish (**1.31**). Food allergic reactions may be IgE-mediated or non-IgE-mediated.

Cow's milk and eggs

Cow's milk and eggs are important allergens in early childhood. The prevalence of documented cow milk allergy is probably no more than 1–2% in the general population, although it may be somewhat higher in early childhood. Cow's milk and egg allergies may cause GI symptoms (such as diarrhoea or vomiting), failure to thrive, skin manifestations (such as maculopapular rash, urticaria or atopic eczema), and localized (lip swelling, angioedema, or laryngeal oedema) or systemic reaction (anaphylaxis). The prognosis is good, since the vast majority of children will lose their allergies to cow's milk and eggs as they grow older.

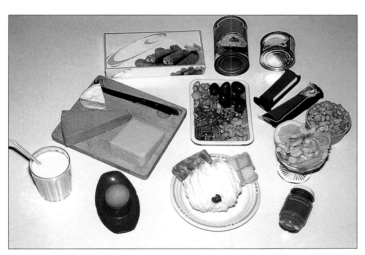

1.31 Common allergenic foods.

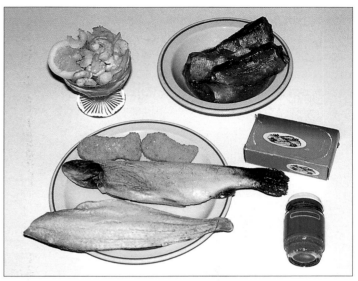

1.32 Fish and shellfish are common food allergens.

Fish and shellfish

Seafoods are composed of diverse sea organisms and many of them cause allergic reactions (**1.32**). Tropomyosin is a major allergen in many shellfish, especially crustacea and molluscs.

Peanuts

Peanuts are the main cause of food-induced anaphylactic reactions. Ara h 1 has been identified as the major peanut allergenic protein. Peanuts (*Arachis hypogaea*) belong to the legume family. However, clinical features of a peanut allergy are more closely related to those of a tree nut allergy, rather than other legumes, such as peas. Peanut allergy occurs in about 0.5–1% of the general population. It is characterized by immediate onset, often with severe symptoms on minimal contact. There is considerable cross-reactivity with one or more tree nuts. Nearly 30% of patients that are allergic to peanuts are also allergic to tree nuts.

Tree nuts

Commonly encountered tree nuts causing allergy include hazelnuts, walnuts, Brazil nuts, almonds, cashews, pecans, chestnuts, pine nuts, pistachios, and coconuts. Allergic reactions to tree nuts can be serious and life-threatening. Attempts have been made to identify and characterize allergenic proteins. Major seed storage proteins include legumins, vicilins, and 2S albumins.

Wheat

Wheat is one of the common allergens, especially in children. Both IgE-mediated and non-IgE-mediated reactions are common. Gliadins are said to be major wheat allergens. IgE antibodies to purified gliadin in children correlate with clinical symptoms on wheat challenge.

Insect allergens

Common insects causing allergic reactions are honeybees, wasps, hornets, yellow jackets, and fire ants. Allergy to bees and wasps occurs in most parts of the world. Reactions may vary from mild localized swelling to systemic reactions and anaphylaxis. Insect stings account for 25% of the cases of severe systemic anaphylaxis referred to an allergy clinic.

Latex

Exposure to latex increased worldwide during the1990s, with a parallel increase in the incidence of latex allergy among the general population, as well as high-risk groups. Latex (natural rubber latex) is encountered widely in rubber-containing products, such as gloves, balloons, catheters, condoms, and surgical instruments (**1.33**). Thus, health care workers and those undergoing frequent surgical procedures have been at high risk. Clinical manifestations include local skin (itching, erythema, oedema, and urticaria), local airways (rhinoconjunctivitis, asthma, and pharyngeal oedema) and/or systemic reactions and, on occasion, anaphylaxis. The use of latex-free gloves and other products has resulted in a significant reduction in incidence of latex allergy.

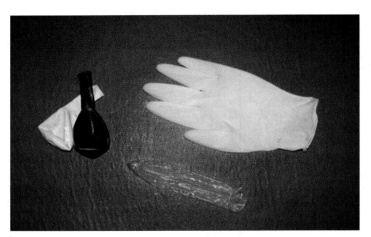

1.33 Commonly used rubber products that may cause allergic reaction in subjects sensitized to natural rubber latex.

Chapter 2

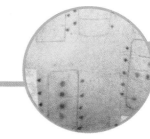

Assessment

Introduction

Diagnosis of allergic diseases is based on clinical criteria, as described in Chapter 1. A comprehensive history and physical examination remains the mainstay of allergy diagnosis, and no single test can confirm or rule out the diagnosis of diseases such as asthma, allergic rhinitis, or AD. However, laboratory tests are useful aids for the diagnosis and, importantly, may help to identify the specific allergen(s) responsible. The outcome of the test should always be interpreted in the light of information available from the clinical assessment.

Table 2.1 outlines some of the tests used in the assessment of allergic disease. These tests can be classified into three groups. *In vitro* tests, such as measurement of specific IgE, are commonly used to confirm allergic status and identify the specific allergen. Other *in vitro* tests, such as blood eosinophil count or basophil histamine release, are rarely helpful and are not commonly used. The second group, *in vivo* or provocation testing, is used extensively for the diagnosis and management of allergic disease. The third group of tests relates to the assessment of environmental exposure to a particular allergen, such as house dust mites or pollen.

Table 2.1 Diagnostic tests

In vitro tests
- Full blood counts
- Total blood eosinophil count
- Sputum and nasal secretion eosinophilia
- Total serum IgE
- Allergen specific IgE
- Radio allergen sorbent test (RAST)
- Competitive RAST inhibition assays
- Allergen specific IgG
- Mast cell tryptase levels
- Basophil histamine release
- Eosinophil cationic protein levels
- Precipitating IgG antibodies
- Exhaled nitric oxide measurements
- Random noise oscillometry

Provocation (in vivo) tests
- Skin tests
- Skin prick tests
- Intradermal skin tests
- Patch testing
- Bronchial and nasal provocation tests
- Food challenge

Assessment of environmental aeroallergens
- Indoor environments
- House dust mite
- Fur-bearing pets (cats, dog, guinea pigs, hamsters)
- Insects (cockroach)
- Moulds

Outdoor environment
- Pollens
- Moulds

Clinical laboratory tests (*in vitro* tests)

Serum total IgE

Serum IgE levels range between 0-0.00001 g/L and approximately 50% of the IgE is localized to the extra-vascular space. The concentration of IgE is age-dependent with cord blood levels being very low. However, atopic infants have a steep rise in their serum IgE during their early years. Extreme elevations of IgE are seen in parasitic infections and hyper-IgE syndrome. A normal or low level of IgE in an asthmatic individual suggests non-IgE mechanisms are playing a role in asthma pathogenesis. In atopic dermatitis, IgE levels are elevated in over 90% of the patients. However, total IgE is not very helpful in the management of allergic diseases. Several immunoassays are available for the measurement of serum total IgE and these include radioimmunoassay (RIA), enzyme linked immuno-sorbent assay (ELISA), and paper radioimmunosorbent assay (PRIST) (**2.1**).

Allergen specific IgE

The presence of allergen-specific IgE is highly indicative of an individual's susceptibility to mount an allergic response upon re-exposure to that allergen. Allergen-specific IgE are assayed using an *in vitro* assay (radio allergen sorbent test, RAST) in serum (**2.2**). RAST measures the amount of IgE that is directed to a specific allergen. Skin tests are generally considered to be more sensitive than RAST assay and it is rare, though not unknown, for a patient to be skin test-negative and RAST-positive. RAST is more expensive than the skin test and results are not available immediately in the clinic. However, RAST may be appropriate in certain situations (*Table 2.2*).

Competitive RAST inhibition assays are used to determine the relative potencies of allergen extracts. One clinical application of RAST inhibition assay has been used as an adjunct to define the appropriate therapeutic

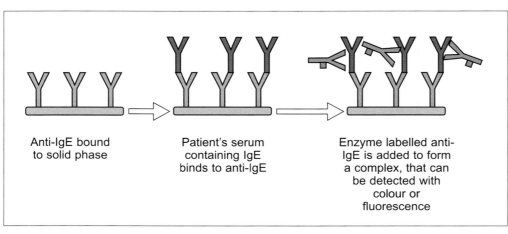

Anti-IgE bound to solid phase

Patient's serum containing IgE binds to anti-IgE

Enzyme labelled anti-IgE is added to form a complex, that can be detected with colour or fluorescence

2.1 Total IgE in blood is often measured using radioimmunoassay.

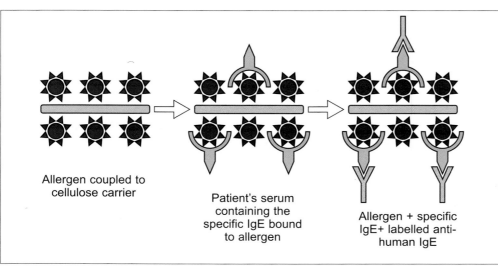

Allergen coupled to cellulose carrier

Patient's serum containing the specific IgE bound to allergen

Allergen + specific IgE+ labelled anti-human IgE

2.2 Serum-specific IgE can be measured *in vitro* by RAST. Several kits are available for measurement of specific IgE to aeroallergens, foods, insect venom, and drugs.

Table 2.2 Indication for radio allergen sorbent test (RAST)

RAST test is indicated:
- Where facilities and/or expertise for a skin test are not available
- When the skin test result is unexpected (e.g. in patients who present with a good history of sensitivity to a particular allergen, and yet produce equivocal or negative skin test results)
- In patients with extensive atopic dermatitis where a large enough area of uninvolved skin is not available
- For subjects who cannot safely discontinue antihistamine (e.g. those with severe allergic rhinitis)
- In patients with extreme sensitivity to food allergens, where there may be a small risk of systemic reaction
- In patients with dermographism
- In epidemiological and clinical research

Table 2.3 Things to remember when performing skin prick test (SPT)

- Always include negative (saline) and positive (histamine) controls
- The prick should be gentle so as not to draw blood
- Care is taken to space individual tests at a sufficient distance from each other so as not to produce overlapping erythema
- Antihistamines should be discontinued 4 days prior to SPT
- Epinephrine and antihistamine should be at hand, but full resuscitation facilities may not be necessary
- Dermatographism can produce false–positive reactions

composition of venoms for patients with hymenoptera sensitivity. These patients, who have potential cross-sensitivities, have opted for immunotherapy.

Mast cell tryptase (MCT)

MCT is a protease that is found in mast cell granules. It is secreted upon stimulation of the cell, together with histamine and many other mediators. Measurement of tryptase in the blood is indicated where there is doubt regarding the nature of a systemic reaction. Tryptase levels are usually, but not always, elevated following an allergic reaction. The assay of tryptase offers significant advantages over other methods of monitoring mast cell activation: it can be performed on serum samples; it is more specific than histamine; and it may be elevated several hours after an allergic reaction.

In vivo tests

Skin prick tests (SPT)

The skin prick or puncture test remains the 'gold standard' in the diagnosis of allergic diseases. It is a biological test for the presence of specific IgE antibodies to the allergen that is being tested (**2.3–2.6**).

Although SPT is a rapid and sensitive test, studies have shown that the reproducibility of the test varies with a coefficient of variation of 15–40%, especially if the wheal diameter is <5 mm. Factors affecting SPT include age (skin reactivity is less in very young and elderly subjects), and concomitant medications, such as antihistamines (*Table 2.3*). SPT is a semi-quantitative test, as the size of the

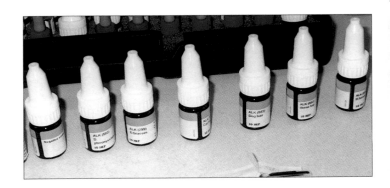

2.3 Extracts are commercially available for a large number of food and aeroallergens.

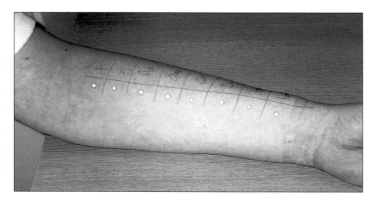

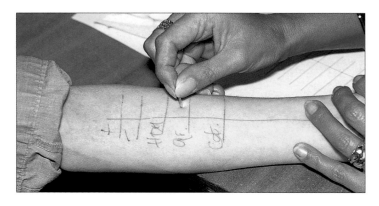

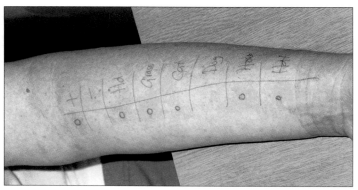

2.4–2.6 SPTs involve placing a drop of allergen extract on the skin of the forearm or back, and introduction of the allergen into the epidermis with a needle puncture. After the prick, the allergen is removed by blotting with a tissue paper. An immediate reaction is read at 15–20 minutes. The longest diameters of the wheal and one perpendicular to it are measured with a millimetre ruler or callipers, and the average is reported. A mean wheal regarded as positive has a diameter of 3 mm greater than the negative control.

Table 2.4 SPT could be graded for semi-quantitative assessment

Grade	Wheal
0	<25% of histamine area
1+	25–50% of histamine area
2+	50–100% of histamine area
3+	100–200% of histamine area
4+	>200% of histamine area

reaction denotes sensitivity of the subject to the specific allergen tested (*Table 2.4*). Sensitization on SPT carries a significant risk for the development of asthma and allergic diseases. The risk increases with increasing number of positive reactions (**2.7–2.9**).

Variation of these tests includes intra-dermal testing which is more sensitive than the standard puncture test. This test requires 0.02 ml of a serial dilution (10–1000-fold) of allergen extract to be injected intra-cutaneously through a 26–27 gauge needle to produce a superficial bleb. Like the skin test, the readings are performed in 15–20 minutes. False–negative reactions can occur when the allergen is injected subcutaneously. Both the wheal and the erythema are measured with a millimetre ruler or calipers. With some dark-skinned people, it is difficult to assess the erythema. Although the reproducibility of the intra-dermal test is better than SPT, this requires greater technical skill. There is also a greater risk of a systemic reaction.

The prick-to-prick test is also used occasionally when allergen extract is either not available or is not reliable, such as when testing for certain fruits. The lancet is pricked in the substance, and the skin is pricked in the same manner as in SPT. The skin reaction is observed and measured.

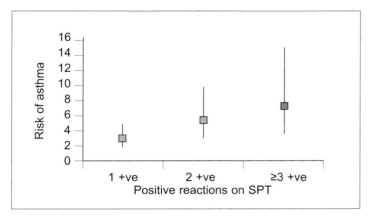

2.7 The risk of asthma (odds ratio and their 95% confidence intervals) in 4-year-old children sensitized to one, two or three or more allergens on SPT.

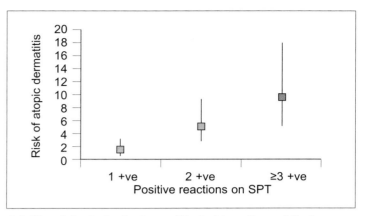

2.8 The risk of atopic dermatitis (odds ratio and their 95% confidence intervals) in 4-year-old children sensitized to one, two, or three or more allergens on SPT.

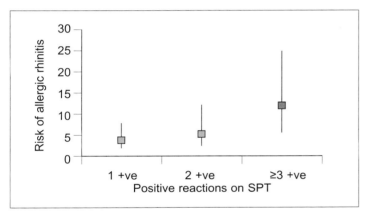

2.9 The risk of allergic rhinitis (odds ratio and their 95% confidence intervals) in 4-year-old children sensitized to one, two, or three or more allergens on SPT.

Patch testing

Patch testing is a way of identifying whether a substance that comes in contact with the skin is causing inflammation of the skin. Patch tests are used for the diagnosis of allergic contact dermatitis. They are indicated in recurrent episodes of contact dermatitis, when needed to identify the offending allergen, and in patients who are not responding to conventional therapy. Patch tests document the presence of delayed-type hypersensitivity (**2.10**).

The test is interpreted as:

- Erythema 1+.
- Oedema or vesicle <50% of patch area 2+.
- Oedema or vesicles >50% of the patch area 3+.

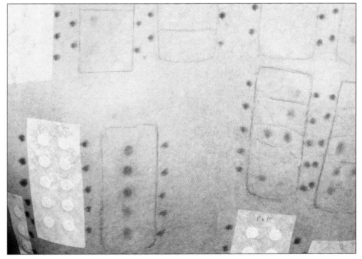

2.10 The allergens are mixed with a non-allergic material (base) to a suitable concentration. They are then placed in direct contact with the skin, usually on the upper back, within small aluminium discs. Adhesive tape is used to fix them in place, and the test sites are marked. The patches are left in place for 48 hours and are usually read at 48 and 72 hours after placement of the allergens.

Systemic corticosteroids and immunosuppressants can suppress the responses. False–positive reactions are due to irritant effect, while false–negatives can occur because the patch tests do not reproduce the exact environment in which the allergen is encountered. Another limitation is the availability of a finite number of allergens.

A range of substances can be used for patch testing. Common substances causing allergic contact dermatitis are included in the European Series Standard Battery (or similar) which is applied to most patients (*Table 2.5*). In addition, other substances can be tested appropriate to the individual circumstances. Each substance has been tested to find the best concentration to demonstrate an allergic reaction without causing irritation to those who are not allergic to the material. Allergens for patch tests are available both in ready-to-use format (**2.11**) and as test material mixed in a vehicle (usually white petroleum).

Bronchial provocation tests

A bronchial provocation test (BPT) is performed to assess quantitatively the state of responsiveness of the airways to allergenic and non-allergenic (non-specific) stimuli. A number of non-allergenic stimuli can be used to provoke bronchi in a standardized manner. These include chemical (histamine, methacholine, bradykinin) and physical stimuli (cold air, exercise). BPTs are commonly used for research purposes, but are clinically useful in the management of patients with cough and wheeze of uncertain cause. Histamine and methacholine are the most commonly used substances. Nebulized histamine or methacholine dissolved in saline is administered through a dosimeter in doubling dilutions. The procedure is stopped if the forced expiratory volume in 1 second (FEV_1) drops by at least 20%, or if the patient becomes symptomatic and is unable to continue the procedure. The degree of airways responsiveness is expressed as PC_{20} the concentration producing a 20% fall in FEV_1 (**2.12**).

This test can also be used to assess bronchial reactivity to allergen (allergen BPT) and to assess the early and late phase responses in patients with allergic asthma. A patient's sensitivity to a particular allergen is first demonstrated on a skin test before that particular allergen is used for allergen BPT. Spirometry is recorded to establish a baseline FEV_1 which should be >70% predicted. After ensuring that the patient is suitable to continue, the subject inhales saline through a dosimeter. The FEV_1 is measured and this value is used to calculate the percentage fall from the post-saline baseline. Following the saline inhalation, the subject inhales varying concentrations of allergen, starting with the least concentration. After each concentration of allergen, a four-fold increment is administered, providing the FEV_1 has not fallen by >10% from the post-saline value. If the fall in FEV_1 is between 10–15%, a two-fold increment is administered. If

Table 2.5 Common chemicals included in the European standard battery

- Nickel sulphate
- Wood alcohols
- Neomycin sulphate
- Potassium dichromate
- Cain mix
- Fragrance mix
- Colophony
- Epoxy resin
- Quinoline mix
- Balsam of Peru
- Ethylenediamine dihydrochloride
- Cobalt chloride
- P-tert-butylphenolformaldehyde
- Paraben mix
- Carba mix
- Black rubber mix
- Kathon CG
- Quaternium-15
- Mercaptobenzothiazole
- p-Phenylenediamine
- Formaldehyde
- Mercapto mix
- Thiomersal
- Thiuram mix

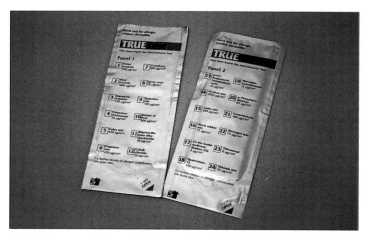

2.11 'True test' is one of the commercially available patch tests that can be easily applied in an office setting.

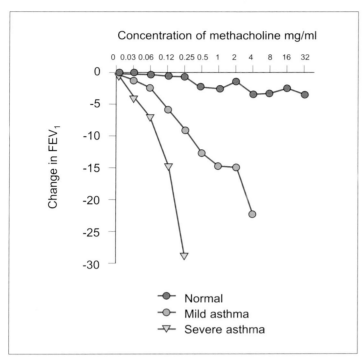

2.12 Methacholine challenge test in normal and asthmatic airways calculates the PC_{20}. Note there is very minimal drop in the FEV_1 in normal individuals, even with 32 mg/ml of methacholine. In severe asthmatics, the 20% drop occurred at 0.25 mg/ml of methacholine.

the fall is >15% but <25% from the post-saline baseline, a dose of the same concentration is administered. The challenge is terminated when a fall in FEV_1 of >25% from the post-saline baseline FEV_1 measurement is achieved. After the final concentration of allergen, FEV_1 measurements are taken at 5, 10, 15, 30, 45, and 60 minutes, and thereafter every 30 minutes up to 10 hours (**2.13**).

Food challenge

A food challenge is performed to confirm or refute the causative relationship of a presumed adverse reaction to a food. It is independent of mechanism, but immediate reactions are suggestive of IgE-mediated food allergy. A food challenge can be open, single blind, or double blind. An open food challenge is easiest to perform, but is subject to bias and is usually not helpful. During a blind food challenge, a patient is given the food to be tested or a placebo, masked in another food or drink to which the patient is not allergic or intolerant. A double blind placebo

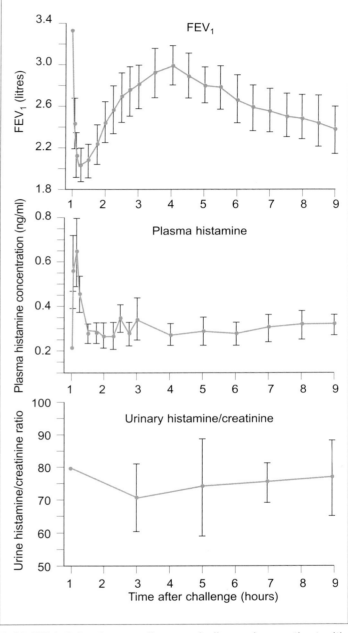

2.13 FEV_1 following an allergen challenge in a patient with allergic asthma shows an early asthmatic response defined as a fall in FEV_1 of at least 25% within 15 minutes of allergen inhalation, and the late asthmatic response defined as a fall in FEV_1 of at least 15% between 3 and 10 hours. The result is expressed as cumulative PD_{20} (provocation dose to cause a 20% fall in FEV_1). Note the early asthmatic response is associated with an increase in the serum histamine levels.

controlled food challenge (DBPCFC) is considered the 'gold standard' in diagnosing food allergy or intolerance. A strict elimination diet of the suspect foods for 7–14 days before the challenge is essential for all types of food challenges. During blind challenges, an equal number of randomly alternating food allergen and placebo challenges are given. The starting dose depends on the sensitivity of the patient (from the history) and the type of food. For example, subjects highly sensitive to nuts may have to have a labial challenge (**2.14**). The dose is gradually increased every 30–60 minutes. Clinical reactivity is ruled out once a substantial amount is given, which is usually the dose that the patient has previously reacted to.

There is no need to undertake a food challenge if a clear-cut history is supplemented by a positive SPT or RAST. Some precautions are recommended, such as avoiding antihistamines, beta 2 agonists, and cromolyn sodium 12 hours prior to the challenge.

Other tests

Sputum induction

Analysis of sputum is useful in assessing the type and degree of airway inflammation. The advantage of induced sputum is that it is inexpensive, safe, and could be performed even in severe asthmatics where bronchoscopy might not be feasible (**2.15**). Studies have shown good correlations with markers of inflammation measured in sputum, broncho-alveolar lavage, and bronchial wash. Though mainly used for research purposes, induced sputum can serve as an excellent tool for the diagnosis of difficult asthma, and to assess the efficacy of treatment (**2.16**).

Fibreoptic bronchoscopy

A bronchoscopy is not a routine test employed in the assessment of allergic airway disease, but serves as a tool to assess the inflammation in airways, and to evaluate the effects of treatment on the inflammatory cell population in the airways. Cytokine levels can also be assayed from bronchoalveolar lavage and bronchial biopsies, to provide clues to the pathophysiologic mechanisms underlying asthma (**2.17**).

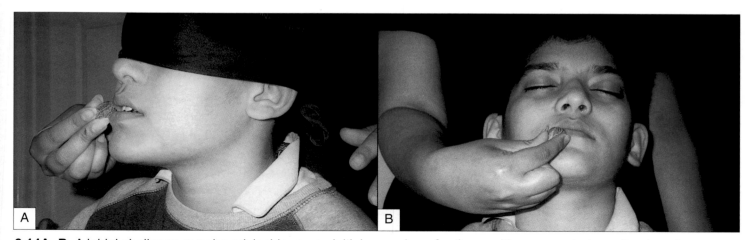

2.14A, B A labial challenge may be advisable, as an initial procedure, for those with a suspected reaction to nuts.

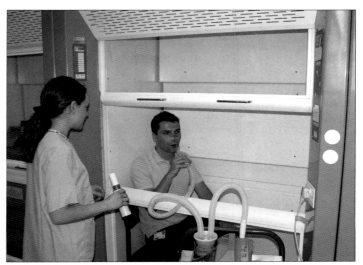

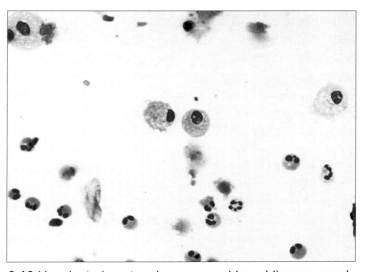

2.15 Sputum induction is carried out using inhaled aerosolized hypertonic saline (4.5%). Subjects are seated in an induction chamber, 400 μg of inhaled salbutamol is administered via a spacer device, and the peak expiratory flow (PEF) is recorded. Patients with a post-bronchodilator FEV_1 of <50% of predicted, and <1.0 L are excluded from the induction procedure for safety reasons. Hypertonic saline is administered via a nebulizer. After every 5 minutes, the nebulization is stopped and PEF measured. The procedure is discontinued when there is a fall in PEF of >15%, or if there are troublesome symptoms. Sputum is expectorated into a Petri dish. The induction period is for a maximum of 20 minutes, or until a satisfactory quality of the sample is obtained.

2.16 Unselected sputum is processed by adding an equal weight of 0.01 M dithioerythritol. The contents are then filtered through a 70 micron filter to remove mucus. The filtrate is centrifuged for 10 minutes at 1500 rpm (400 g) at 40°C to pellet the cells. The cell pellet is re-suspended in 1 ml of tris-buffered saline and cells are counted in a Neubauer's chamber after staining with trypan blue. Cytospins are obtained based on the total cell counts, and the cells are stained by Rapi-Diff stain. The figure shows sputum eosinophilia in severe asthma. Eosinophils show bilobed nuclei with pink cytoplasm. The capability of eosinophils to degranulate and release biologically active lipids enables them to contribute to the immunopathogenesis of asthma and rhinitis.

2.17 Bronchoscopy is performed using a fibreoptic bronchoscope. The subject fasts for 5 hours prior to bronchoscopy and is premedicated with nebulized salbutamol (2.5 mg) and intra-venous atropine (0.6 mg). Light sedation is achieved with intra-venous midazolam (0–6 mg). Topical 10% lignocaine spray is used for local anaesthesia (total maximum lignocaine dose <300 mg). Oxygen saturation is monitored throughout the procedure by pulse oximetry. Bronchial biopsies are taken from the subcarinae of the 2nd- and 3rd-generation bronchi of the right lower lobe (using alligator forceps), and are placed in a tissue culture medium for subsequent microscopic examination or culture studies, or are processed into glycol methacrylate resin for immunohistochemistry analysis. Bronchial washings and lavage may also yield useful information.

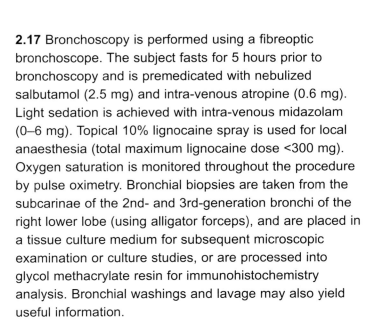

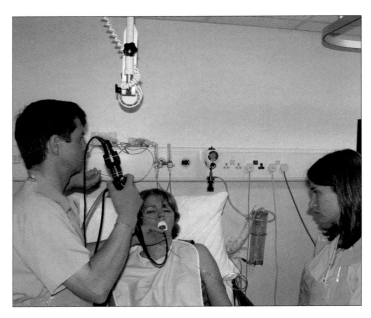

Endobronchial ultrasound

Endobronchial ultrasound is a technique used in research to evaluate the thickness of the airway mucosa in asthma. It is useful in improving the diagnostic yield with transbronchial needle aspiration and transbronchial lung biopsies. However, its use as a research tool in asthma is still at a very early stage (**2.18**).

Nitric oxide (NO)

Nitric oxide is an inorganic, gaseous free radical that carries a variety of messages between cells. Vasorelaxation, neurotransmission, and cytotoxicity can all be potentiated through cellular response to NO. The formation of NO is catalysed by inducible NO synthase (iNOS). Cytokines, such as INF-γ, TNF, IL-1 and IL-2, and lipopolysaccharides, cause an increase in iNOS messenger ribonucleic acid (mRNA), protein, and activity levels. Protein kinase C stimulating agents exhibit the same effect on iNOS activity. After cytokine induction, iNOS exhibits a delayed activity response, which is then followed by a significant increase in NO production over a long period of time. NO, *per se*, can exert damaging effects on cells or could react with superoxide to form peroxynitrite, a powerful oxidant capable of exerting cytotoxic effects. NO also plays a role in regulating the immune response and can inhibit lymphocyte proliferation.

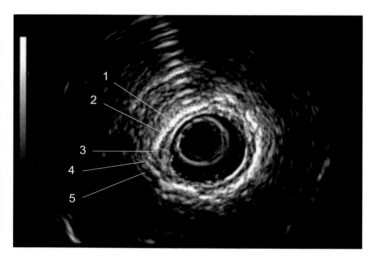

2.18 An endobronchial ultrasound showing cross-section of a bronchus. (1, first hyperechoic band: marginal echo from mucosa/submucosa; 2, second hypoechoic band: mucosa/submucosa; 3, third hyperechoic band: internal edge of cartilage; 4, fourth hypoechoic band: cartilage; 5, fifth hyperechoic band: external edge of cartilage/adventitia.) (Courtesy of Dr TJ Shaw, Southampton General Hospital, Southampton, UK.)

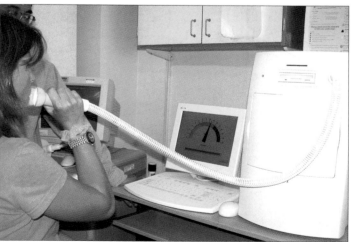

2.19 NO in exhaled breath is a simple, quick, and non-invasive test that may find a place in the clinical management of asthma.

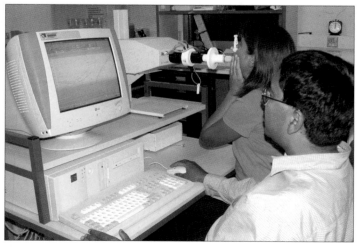

2.20 Forced oscillation technique offers simple, quick, non-invasive, and patient-friendly measurement of airflow obstruction.

NO levels are found to be elevated in acute asthma and these levels drop significantly following treatment with corticosteroids. Hence, it is a useful surrogate marker for airway inflammation and could be used to monitor the response to treatment (**2.19**). However, exhaled NO is not specific for asthma, and its levels have been shown to be elevated in adult respiratory distress syndrome (ARDS) and pneumonias.

Forced oscillation technique

Forced oscillation technique is a relatively new technique used to asses the lung function. It measures the airway resistance which indicates the degree of airflow obstruction. During the test, patients have tidal breathing against the oscillatory wave (4–30 Hz) produced by a Pseudo Random Noise Oscillometer, and the impedance of the airway is calculated (**2.20**).

Potentially, there are several advantages of the forced oscillation technique. As it requires only passive co-operation, it could be done in infants, children, severe asthmatics, and elderly patients for whom traditional spirometry might be difficult. Furthermore, as this test is done during tidal breathing, it is more physiological and eliminates the problems associated with forced expiratory manoeuvres. Thus, it may provide a more reliable means of measuring lung function. In addition, this technique offers the potential to study resistance in large and small airways independently of each other.

Assessment of environmental allergens

Indoor allergens

Allergen avoidance forms an important aspect of management of allergic diseases. The assessment of exposure to a specific allergen may indicate the level of risk and the need to implement avoidance measures. Predominant indoor allergens include house dust mites, cockroaches, animal dander, and moulds. These allergens can be measured in the house dust collected with a dust collector.

Standardized protocols are available for dust collections, for example, sampling of 1 m² of mattress or carpet which is vacuumed for 1 or 2 minutes. The collected dust is sieved to remove hair, fluff, and large particles. Major allergens from these sources can be measured in the fine dust with the results commonly reported as µg or ng/g of dust. Quantitative analysis of the indoor environment enables assessment of individual risks in sensitized patients in a particular home, and to monitor the effects of environmental control (**2.21**). Levels of house dust mite major allergens (*Der p and Der f*) of 2 and 10 µg/g of dust have been suggested as indicating risk for sensitization and development of asthmatic symptoms.

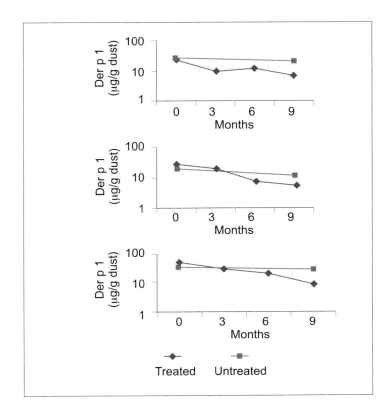

2.21 Repeated application of Acarosan®, an anti-dust mite spray (based on benzyl benzoate) led to the reduction in the level of dust mite allergens in the treated group. (Adapted from Arshad HS *et al.* [1992]. Effect of food and house-dust mite allergen avoidance on development of allergic disorders in infancy. *Lancet*, **339**:1493–97.)

Outdoor allergens

Outdoor allergens include pollens and moulds. Pollen (tree, grass, and weed) in the air is sampled through a pollen trap (**2.22**) at different locations in the country. Pollen and mould levels are reported in grains or spores per cubic meter of air sampled for the previous 24-hour period. During the pollen season, between March and September, pollen count is monitored daily in the UK by the environmental agencies and the information is provided to the general public. This can also serve to devise the pollen calendar for particular regions (**2.23**). This calendar is useful for patients with seasonal allergic rhinoconjunctivitis who need to take appropriate precautions to reduce exposure on days when the pollen count is high.

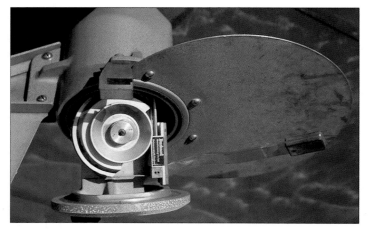

2.22 Pollen trap. Air is sucked through a narrow slit on the side of the pollen trap and lands on a sticky tape or glass slide. Pollen and other particles in the air stick to the tape or glass surface. The tape/slide is taken off and pollen counting is done under the light microscope.

Taxa	January	February	March	April	May	June	July	August	September
Hazel (*Corylus*)									
Yew (*Taxus*)									
Alder (*Alnus*)									
Alm (*Ulmus*)									
Willow (*Salix*)									
Poplar (*Populus*)									
Birch (*Betula*)									
Ash (*Fraxinus*)									
Plane (*Platanus*)									
Oak (*Quercus*)									
Oil seed rape (*B. napus*)									
Pine (*Pinus*)									
Grass (*Gramineae*)									
Plantain (*Plantago*)									
Lime (*Tilia*)									
Nettle (*Urtica*)									
Dock (*Rumex*)									
Mugwort (*Artemisia*)									

——— Main period of pollen release

——— Peak periods

2.23 Pollen calendar for the UK. (Adapted from data from The National Pollen and Aerobiology Research Unit, University College Worcester, Worcester, UK.)

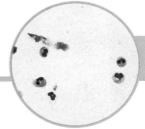

Chapter 3

Asthma

Epidemiology

The prevalence of asthma has increased to epidemic proportions, and the current health care expenditure for asthma in the industrialized countries is enormous. In Western Europe, asthma has doubled in the last 10 years, and in the US it has increased by over 60% since the 1980s. The human and economic burden associated with asthma is large and the economic cost is estimated to exceed that of tuberculosis and HIV/AIDS combined together. It is an irony that 43% of the cost of asthma care is related to the use of emergency departments in hospitals. The International Study of Asthma and Allergies in Childhood (ISAAC) looked at the prevalence and severity of asthma, rhinitis, and eczema in children living in different centres to help make comparisons within and between countries. The mean prevalence of any wheeze in the past 12 months ranged from under 5% in Albania, China, Greece, Georgia, Indonesia, Romania, and Russia to 29–32% in Australia, New Zealand, Republic of Ireland, and the UK (**3.1**). The prevalence of four or more attacks, which is a more specific indicator of clinically important asthma, ranged from <1% in Albania, Indonesia, Uzbekistan, Russia, Romania, Greece, Georgia, and China to over 9% in Australia, New Zealand, UK, and Canada. These rates of prevalence tended to correlate with those of less frequent wheezing. This suggests that higher prevalences of wheezing in these English-speaking countries are unlikely to be explained solely by over-reporting of mild symptoms. Studies in adults show similar variation (**3.2**).

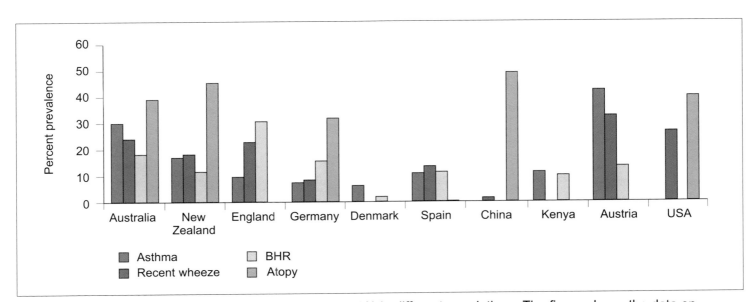

3.1 The prevalence of asthma symptoms varies from 0–30% in different populations. The figure shows the data on prevalence of diagnosed asthma, recent wheeze, bronchial hyper-responsiveness (BHR), and atopy in children. (Data adapted from the ISAAC study. Asthma, GIF [2002]. *Global Strategy for Asthma Management and Prevention*, National Institute of Health: a1–1176.)

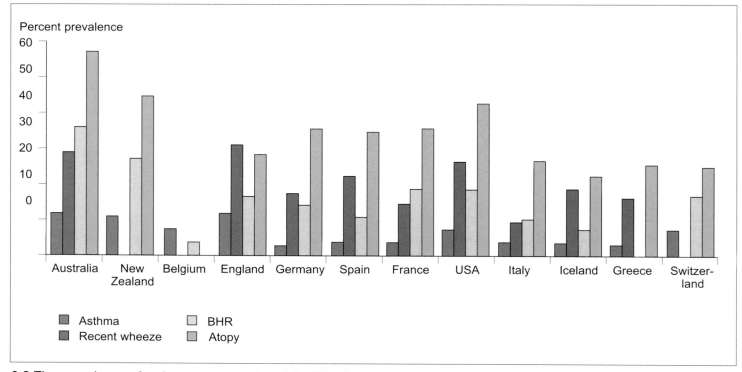

3.2 The prevalence of asthma symptoms in adults. The figure shows the data on prevalence of diagnosed asthma, recent wheeze, bronchial hyper-responsiveness (BHR), and atopy in adults. (Data adapted from studies in the Australian population and the European Community Respiratory Health Survey (ECRHS). Asthma, GIF [2002]. *Global Strategy for Asthma Management and Prevention*, National Institute of Health: a1–1176.)

Development and risk factors

Both host and environmental factors affect the risk of development of asthma (**3.3**). Atopy is the strongest risk factor, increasing the risk by 10–20-fold, compared with those who are non-atopic. The level of IgE is associated with the prevalence and severity of bronchial hyper-responsiveness (BHR) and asthma. However, asthma is non-atopic in nearly half of older children and adults, and important susceptibility genes may be inherent to the airway wall (**3.4**).

Most asthma originates in the early stages of life (**3.5**). Childhood asthma tends to be a predominantly male disease. After 20 years of age, the prevalence remains approximately equal until age 40, when the disease becomes more common in females. Abnormal BHR is a central feature of asthma. However, not all patients with BHR have symptoms of asthma. BHR frequently precedes, and is associated with, an elevated risk for wheeze onset and recurrent asthma in adolescents.

Exposure to dust mites within the first year of life is associated with later development of asthma, and possibly atopy (**3.6**). Inhalation of cigarette smoke during pregnancy has been linked with abnormal lung functions, BHR, and allergy in the newborn. Tobacco smoke is also an important trigger factor for asthma attacks. Some recent studies have shown a relationship between passive smoking and the development of asthma. In addition, air pollution plays a well-documented role in asthma attacks. Ozone is a key player in the development and aggravation of asthma. The 'hygiene hypothesis' suggests that lack of exposure to a childhood infection, endotoxin, and bacterial products are important determinants regarding development of atopic disease. Environmental exposure to microbial antigens and bacterial compounds helps the development of immune tolerance through the stimulation of Th1 cells and/or suppression of Th2 cells, preventing the development of allergic disorders in children.

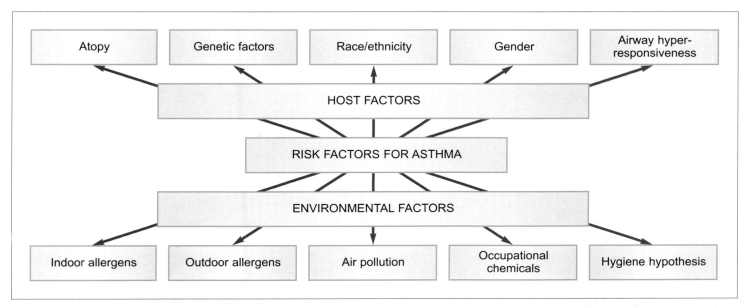

3.3 Asthma is a heterogeneous disease with various factors including the environment, genetics, levels of hygiene, and atopic status playing a role in its development and progression.

3.4 Gene–environment interactions in the development of asthma and atopy. By separating local tissue susceptibility factors from those that predispose to the development of atopy, this scheme shows how atopy can develop in the absence of asthma and how the allergic predisposition can interact with airway susceptibility factors to promote the asthmatic phenotype. (ETS, environmental tobacco smoke.) (Adapted from Davies DE *et al.* [2003]. Airway remodeling in asthma: new insights. *J Allergy Clin Immunol*, **111(2)**:215–25.)

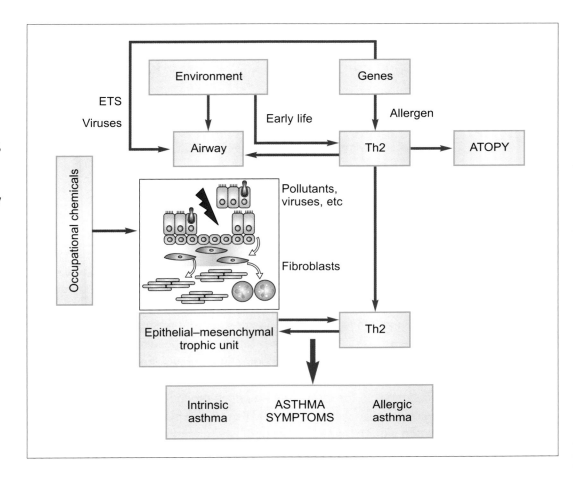

Pathophysiology

In predisposed individuals, exposure to allergen results in an early response starting within minutes after an allergen challenge. In 50–80% of patients this is followed by a late response. The early reaction is thought to be a reflection of mast cell degranulation, while the late response reflects the multi-cellular events more analogous to the inflammatory response seen in asthma (**3.7**). One of the distinguishing features of asthma is the presence of BHR. This increased

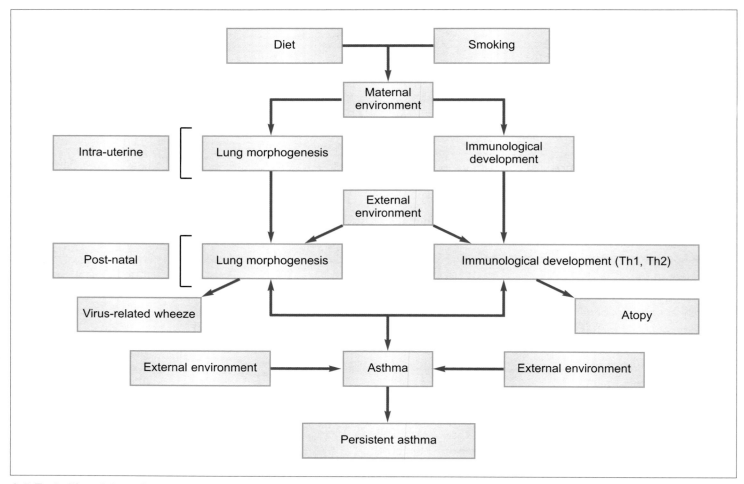

3.5 Early life origins of asthma. The first symptoms of asthma can occur at any age, but recurrent episodes of wheezing and airway obstruction manifest before 6 years of age in most patients. Genetic factors include cytokine dysregulation with a tendency toward Th2 responses, or a deficiency of Th1 activity, either of which would promote allergy sensitization. Environmental factors include infections, allergen exposure, and pollutants. The development of allergic asthma can be considered as a two-stage process. The first stage involves the development of allergen-specific immunological memory against inhaled allergens. This happens in childhood and polarizes the immune response towards a Th2 phenotype. These individuals are therefore more prone to develop allergic inflammation. The predisposition to allergic airway disease could be due to the differences in the intra-uterine priming process. There is evidence to suggest that the materno-foetal interface is immunologically active with a predominance of Th2 cytokines. In non-atopic individuals, the initial low level Th2 immunity is converted into Th1 during childhood, whereas the process fails in atopics, leading to the consolidation of Th2 polarized response. Stage 2 involves consolidation and maintenance of these polarized Th2 responses leading to a state of chronic airway inflammation. This second phase is influenced by various factors, such as respiratory viral infections, repeated indoor and outdoor allergen exposure, environmental tobacco smoke, and air pollutants. (Adapted from Davies DE *et al.* [2003]. Airway remodeling in asthma: new insights. *J Allergy Clin Immunol*, **111(2)**:215–25.)

airway responsiveness to various triggers is associated with an underlying inflammatory process in the large and small airways.

The airway wall thickness is increased in asthma and is related to the severity (**3.8**). Compared to non-asthmatic subjects, the airway wall thickness is increased from 50–300% in cases of fatal asthma and from 10–100% in cases of non-fatal asthma. The increase in thickness is due

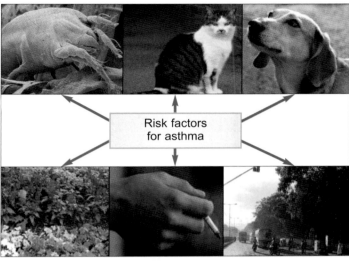

3.6 Environmental exposure in sensitized individuals is a major contributor to the development of asthma.

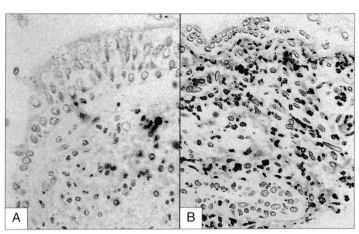

3.7 Allergen challenge induces recruitment of eosinophils into the airways. The photomicrograph (**A**) shows an asthmatic bronchial biopsy stained for eosinophils by immunohistochemistry. Panel **B** shows the same subject after inhalation of allergen. Note the increase in the number of eosinophils in the bronchial biopsy following allergen challenge.

3.8 Transmission electron micrograph of a section of airway wall with corresponding illustrations. Bronchial epithelium consisting of ciliated and secretory columnar epithelial cells (1) and basal cells (2) bound to a basement membrane (3). The basement membrane separates the epithelium from the submucosa (4). Contact with inhaled material occurs at the ciliated apical surface of the columnar cells. The panel on the left is a section of normal airways, and the panel on the right

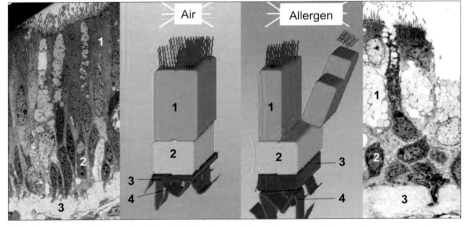

is from asthmatic airways. Note the shedding of columnar cells and cilia, thickening of the basement membrane, and increase in smooth muscle in the submucosa. Epithelial damage is a characteristic feature of asthma. The epithelial damage and shedding occurs as a consequence of separation of the columnar cells from the basal cells, which are more resistant to detachment in asthma even in the presence of extensive inflammation. The damage to the epithelium due to the constant insult is accompanied by increased repair resulting in a steady state that probably never allows complete healing. (Reprinted from Holgate S [2003]. Pathology of asthma in 'Asthma: definitions and pathogenesis', *Allergy: Principles and Practice,* 6th edn, Mosby, pp1177–80, with permission from Elsevier Ltd.)

to increase in most tissue compartments including: smooth muscle, epithelium, submucosa, adventitia, and mucosal glands. The inflammatory oedema involves the whole airways, particularly the submucosal layer with marked hypertrophy and hyperplasia of the submucosal glands, and goblet cell hyperplasia. Goblet cell hyperplasia and hypertrophy is a non-specific response to the loss of epithelial cells, and this is particularly evident in the smaller airways of patients with fatal asthma (**3.9**). There is hyperplasia of the muscularis layer, and microvascular vasodilatation in the adventitial layers of the airways. This increased wall thickness will amplify the effects of smooth muscle shortening on airway narrowing, and the effect is in direct relation to the degree of the airway wall thickness. The airway pathology in asthma is characterized by: an increase in smooth muscle mass; mucous gland hypertrophy and hyperplasia; persistence of chronic inflammatory cellular infiltrates; epithelial damage leading to airway narrowing; and obstruction due to mucous plugs (**3.10**).

The inflammatory infiltrate in asthma is multi-cellular in nature and characteristically involves T-cells, eosinophils, neutrophils, macrophages/monocytes, and mast cells (**3.11**). Airway inflammation leads to repair mechanisms being put into place. Airway inflammation and remodelling are intensively intertwined in their end-result of lung function loss and airway hyper-responsiveness (AHR). Inflammatory cells mainly influence airway wall remodelling by production of mediators that either directly induce structural cells to proliferate and/or produce matrix components, or indirectly affect structural cells by stimulation of other local cells (**3.12**). Epithelial shedding in asthma is a characteristic feature that is not observed in other inflammatory diseases (**3.13**). Epithelial damage is accompanied by profibrogenic growth factors. Among these growth factors, TGF-β is particularly important because it promotes differentiation of fibroblasts into myofibroblasts that secrete interstitial collagens. This communication between the epithelium and mesenchymal cells is reminiscent of the modelling of the airways during embryonic development, and has led to the hypothesis that the epithelial–mesenchymal trophic unit remains activated after birth, or becomes reactivated in asthma and drives the remodelling of the asthmatic airways (**3.14, 3.15**).

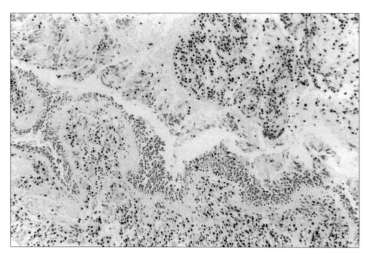

3.9 Bronchial biopsy showing a predominance of eosinophils in the submucosa in a fatal asthmatic.

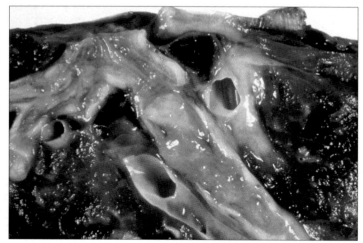

3.10 Mucous plug causing airway obstruction in a case of fatal asthma. The characteristic mucous plugs of the asthmatic airways cause airway obstruction leading to ventilation–perfusion mismatch, contributing to hypoxemia which cannot be compensated by hyperventilation. This thick and tenacious mucous plug extends to the membranous bronchiole, with the plugs often being continuous with mucus in the ducts and lumen of the submucosal glands. Mucous plugs are composed of mucus, serum proteins, inflammatory cells, and cellular debris which includes desquamated epithelial cells and macrophages often arranged in a spiral pattern (Curshmann's spirals). The excessive mucus production in fatal asthma is attributed to hypertrophy and hyperplasia of the submucosal glands.

3.11 Bronchial biopsy stained for mast cells in a subject with asthma. Mast cells are important effector cells in asthma, and have a key role in the early phase asthmatic response.

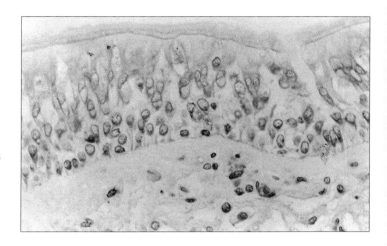

3.12 Bronchial epithelial cells are activated in asthma as shown by the increased expression of membrane markers such as ICAM-1 or HLA-DR, and an increased spontaneous release of pro-inflammatory mediators. Endothelin-1 influences the airway caliber, and its expression has been found in the epithelium of the airways of asthmatics, but not in normal subjects. Epithelial injury leads to a complex series of repair mechanisms. Bronchial epithelial cells can be directly triggered by allergens and not growth. Lastly, viruses can directly damage epithelial cells. Inflammatory mediators, such as histamine, platelet activating factor, or cytokines, can also activate bronchial epithelial cells. Remodelling of the airways in asthma involves structural changes in the epithelium, the myofibroblasts, and extra-cellular matrix (including basement membrane), and smooth muscle. This remodelling process is mainly orchestrated by a complex interaction of inflammatory cells (central in the pathogenesis of asthma), with structural tissue cells. Once present, airway remodelling may contribute to the chronic nature of airway inflammation.

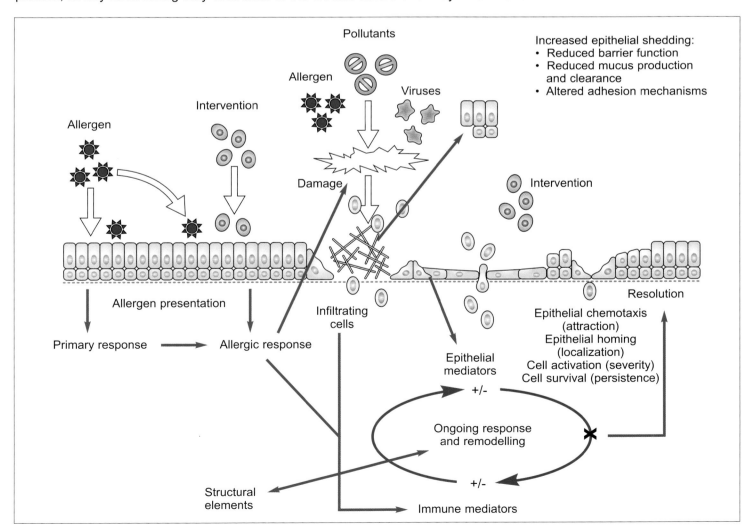

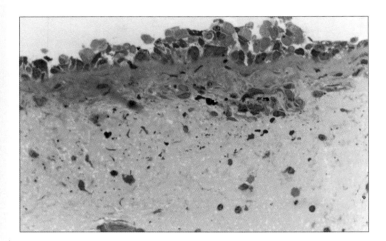

3.13 Bronchial epithelium in an asthmatic showing epithelial damage and shedding. Epithelial shedding and epithelial damage correlate with bronchial hyper-reactivity (toluidine blue staining).

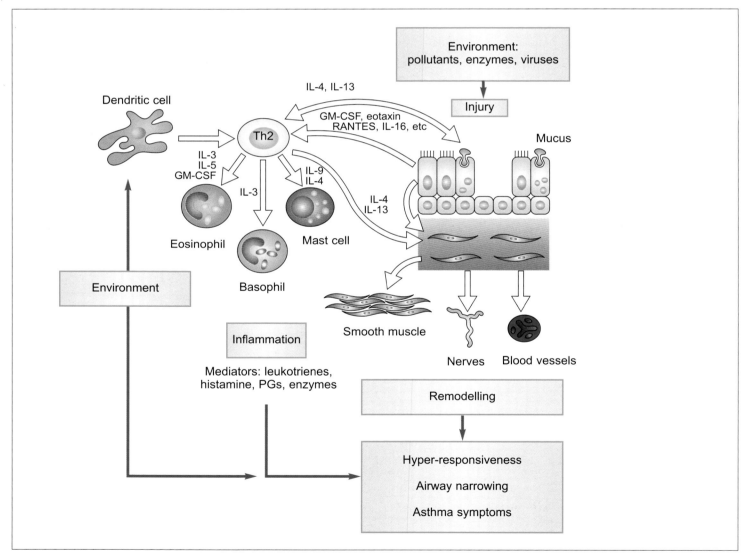

3.14 Airway inflammation and remodelling occur simultaneously, as a result of immune-related damage, causing airway narrowing and bronchial hyper-responsiveness. (GM-CSF, granulocyte monocyte colony stimulting factor; IL, interleukin; PG, prostaglandin.)

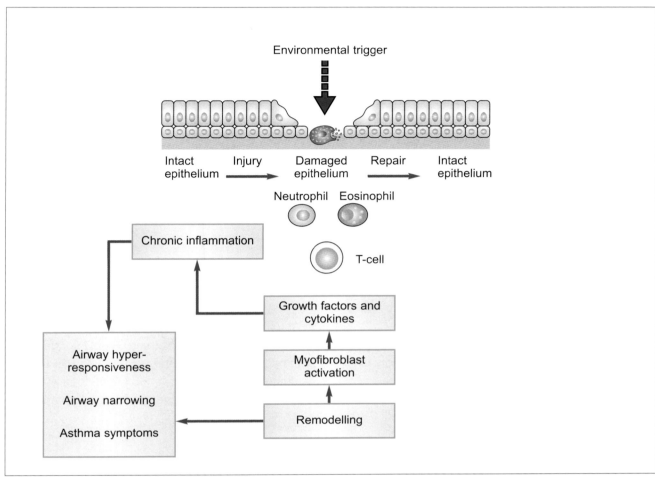

3.15 Following epithelial damage, repair mechanisms come in play restoring intact epithelium, but also causing mesenchymal proliferation with consequent airway remodelling.

Clinical features

It is essential to be as certain as possible of a primary diagnosis of asthma. This rests on a clinical history, physiological evidence of variable and reversible airway obstruction, and exclusion of a possible alternative diagnosis that may mimic asthma. Objective evidence of asthma includes variability of peak flows and FEV_1 (**3.16**). Most patients with asthma will show a variability of at least 20% in peak expiratory flow rate (PEFR) (**3.17**). Reversibility of airway obstruction after inhalation of a short-acting beta 2 agonist is highly suggestive of asthma. Lung function tests and flow–volume loops can be useful to rule out other diagnoses (**3.18, 3.19**). Challenge testing with histamine or methacholine is not routinely used for the diagnosis, but can serve as a useful tool in patients with a doubtful diagnosis (**3.20**). Sputum eosinophilia is a feature of asthma; however, recent studies have shown that a subset of patients with severe asthma have a predominance of neutrophils rather than eosinophils in their sputum (**3.21, 3.22**).

Acute exacerbations of asthma are episodes of shortness of breath, cough, and wheezing associated with chest tightness. These attacks are characterized by reduction in the PEFR and FEV_1. The intensity of asthma exacerbations may vary from mild, to moderate, to severe (*Table 3.1*, p46). Among patients attending the emergency department, the severity of obstruction in terms of FEV_1 is on average 30–35% of predicted. Patients are dyspnoeic at rest, and are

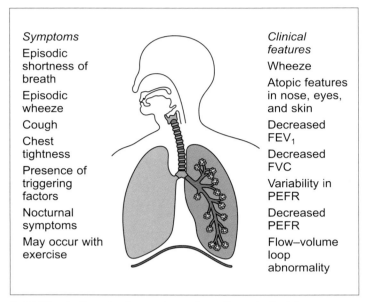

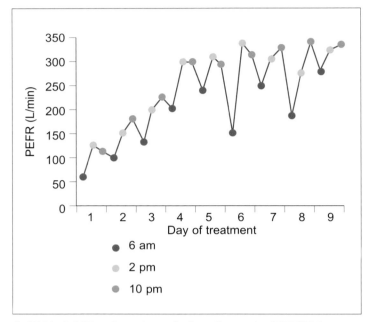

3.16 The hallmark of symptoms in asthma is that they are variable, intermittent, worse at night, and provoked by various triggering factors. Other information contributing to the diagnosis of asthma include a positive family history of allergy or asthma, and worsening symptoms after taking non-steroidal anti-inflammatory drugs, aspirin, or beta blockers. (FEV$_1$, forced expiratory volume in 1 second; FVC, forced vital capacity; PEFR, peak expiratory flow rate.)

3.17 Variability of peak expiratory flow rate (PEFR) is a characteristic feature of asthma. Highly suggestive of asthma is a 20% or greater variability in PEFR, with a minimum change of at least 60 L/min, ideally for 2 days in a week for 2 weeks, seen over a period of time.

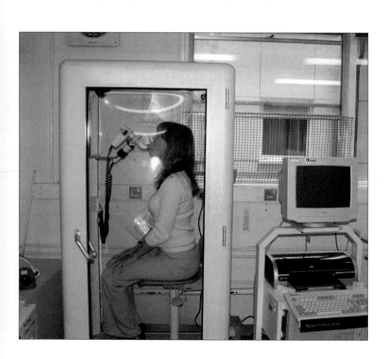

3.18 A whole body plethysmograph is used to estimate the volumes of the lungs. The body box is a sealed chamber, in which the patient sits and breathes through a tube passing out of the box. Since the volume of the patient will change during the breathing cycle, the air pressure inside the box will vary. The residual volume within the lungs can be found by measuring the pressure in the airways when the patient tries to inhale from a closed tube. The residual volume can then be calculated from the increased volume of the lungs and the reduced pressure during attempted inspiration. The body box is more useful for testing children, since spirometry results are effort dependent. The body box can measure the specific airway resistance (sRaw) in children, and can provide useful information in asthma. Furthermore, the lung volume measurements can differentiate between asthma and emphysema.

3.19 The flow–volume loop is generated by continuously recording flow and volume. The shape of the loop reflects the status of the lung volumes and airways throughout the respiratory cycle. Characteristic changes occur in restrictive disorders, as well as in obstructive ones. The loop is especially helpful in detecting laryngeal and tracheal lesions. Airway obstruction is indicated by the overall concave shape of the upper part of the graph.

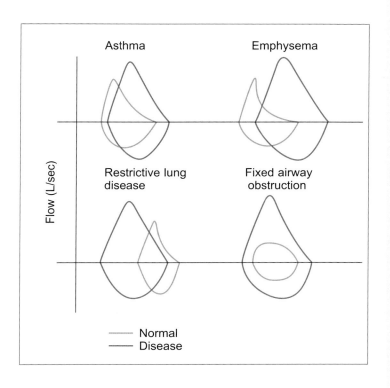

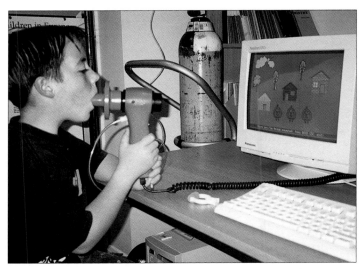

3.20 Methacholine bronchial challenge being performed on a patient.

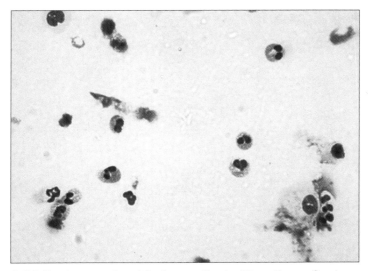

3.21 Sputum eosinophils in a patient with asthma. Sputum eosinophilia is a characteristic feature of asthma.

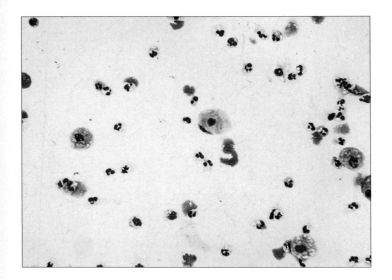

3.22 In severe asthma, there is a predominance of neutrophils in the sputum, as seen in this specimen from a patient with severe corticosteroid dependent asthma. Neutrophilic inflammation is of clinical relevance, because it is associated with nocturnal asthma, oral steroid dependent asthma, and chronic severe asthma.

Table 3.1 Asthma severity varies widely in patients at the doctor's office or emergency departments

Factors	Mild	Moderate	Severe	Imminent respiratory arrest
Breathlessness	Walking	Talking	At rest	Drowsy/confused
Talks in	Sentences	Phrases	Words	
Alertness	Agitation ±	Usually agitated	Usually agitated	
Accessory muscles and supra-sternal retractions	Usually not	Usually	Usually	Abdominal paradox
Wheeze	End-expiratory	Throughout expiration	Inspiratory and expiratory	Absent
Pulse	<100 bpm	100–120 bpm	>120 bpm	Bradycardia
Respiratory rate	Increased	Increased	>30/minute	Absent
Pulsus paradox	<10 mmHg	10–25 mmHg	>25 mmHg	
PEFR	>80%	60–80%	<60% or <100 L/min	
PaO_2	Normal	>60 mmHg	<60 mmHg	
SaO_2	>95%	91–95%	<90%	
$PaCO_2$	<45 mmHg	<45 mmHg	>45 mmHg	

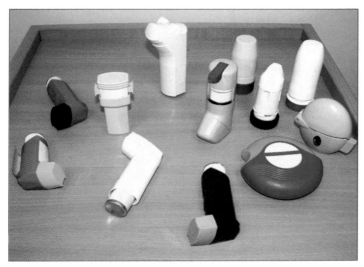

3.23 Inhalers in asthma.

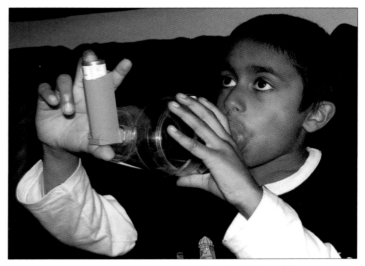

3.24 A patient using a metered dose inhaler with a spacer device.

unable to complete sentences or phrases. Wheeze can be heard both during inspiration and expiration. They are agitated in the early stages, and drowsiness and confusion are ominous signs. The respiratory rate is high and the patient usually sits upright using accessory muscles of respiration to aid in breathing.

Physical examination should also look for the presence of complications including pneumothorax, subcutaneous emphysema, atelectasis, pneumonia, and evidence of theophylline toxicity.

Treatment

The aims of pharmacological management of asthma are clearly described in most guidelines (*Table 3.2*). Asthma medications are generally divided into relievers and controllers. Controllers are medications taken daily on a long-term basis that are useful in getting and keeping persistent asthma under control (*Table 3.3*). Medications for asthma have various forms of administration, including inhaled, oral (ingested), and parenteral (subcutaneous, intramuscular, or intravenous). The major advantage of delivering drugs directly into the airways via inhalation is that high concentrations can be delivered more effectively to the airways, and systemic side-effects are avoided or minimized. Some of the drugs that are effective in asthma can only be used via inhalation because they are not absorbed when given orally (e.g. anticholinergics and

Table 3.2 Goals of asthma therapy

- Maintain normal activity levels
- Maintain normal pulmonary function
- Prevent chronic symptoms
- Prevent recurrent exacerbations
- Provide optimal pharmacotherapy with least side-effects

cromones). The onset of action of bronchodilators is substantially quicker when they are given via inhalation than when these drugs are administered orally. Aerosolized medications that are used to treat asthma are available as pressurized metered-dose inhalers (MDIs), breath-actuated MDIs, dry powder inhalers (DPIs), and nebulized medications (**3.23**). The use of a volumatic chamber provides added advantages, such as reducing the amount of drugs deposited in the oropharynx (thereby reducing the adverse affects), better delivery of the medications to the airways, and reducing the incidence of cough following inhalation (**3.24**).

Table 3.3 Dosages of long-term asthma medications

Medication	Adult dose	Child dose	Side-effects
Systemic corticosteroids			
Methyl prednisolone	7.5–60 mg/day	0.25–2 mg/kg/day	Bruising, thinning of skin, occasional adrenal suppression, minor growth delay or suppression in children. Long-term use can cause osteoporosis, hypertension, cataracts, obesity, muscle weakness
Prednisolone	40–60 mg/day	1–2 mg/kg/day	
Long-acting beta 2 agonist			
Salmeterol	50 µg twice daily	50 µg twice daily	Anxiety, tachycardia, muscle tremor, hypokalaemia
Formoterol	12 µg twice daily	12 µg twice daily	
Cromones			
Cromolin sodium	1 mg/puff; 2–4 puffs 3–4 times a day	1–2 puffs 3–4 times a day	Cough on inhalation
Nedocromil sodium	1.75 mg/puff; 2–4 puffs 3–4 times a day	1–2 puffs 3–4 times a day	
Leukotriene modifiers			
Montelukast	10 mg once daily	4 mg once daily (2–5 yrs)	Reversible hepatitis, deranged liver enzymes, unmasking of Churgg–Strauss syndrome
Zafirlukast	20 mg twice daily	10 mg daily (7–11 yrs)	
Zileuton	600 mg 4 times a day	–	
Methylxanthines			
Theophylline	10 mg/kg/day	10 mg/kg/day >1 year 16 mg/kg/day	Nausea, vomiting, tachycardia, arrhythmias and seizures
Inhaled corticosteroids			
Beclomethasone CFC			Local effects such as oropharyngeal candidiasis and hoarseness of voice. High doses can cause skin thinning and bruising, and suppression or growth delay in children
Beclomethasone HFC			
Budesonide			
Flunisolide			
Fluticasone			
Triamcinalone acetonide			

Inhaled corticosteroids need to be administered on an individual basis because asthmatics differ in their needs and tolerances. The dosage also depends on the severity of the asthma, which varies over time. Each generic drug type varies in strength and effectiveness. Inhaled steroids are best given on a twice-daily basis. A common starting dose is between 100–400 µg. High doses of 600–2000 µg may be necessary to gain control of severe asthma. Usually a low dose is started with, and the dose is increased until the asthma stabilizes

A comprehensive plan of asthma management should consider all possible options, including allergen avoidance, patient education, pharmacotherapy, and allergen-specific immunotherapy (**3.25**). Although there is no cure, treatment for asthma aims at providing adequate control with minimal side-effects. This is achieved by a stepwise approach to asthma management. The presence of symptoms at night or early in the morning, and measurement of PEFR and its variability, are helpful in the initial assessment of asthma severity and in monitoring the initial treatment. It is also helpful in assessing changes in severity and preparing for a reduction in therapy (*Table 3.4*, p50). In the stepwise approach to therapy, progression to the next step is indicated when control is not achieved or is lost with the

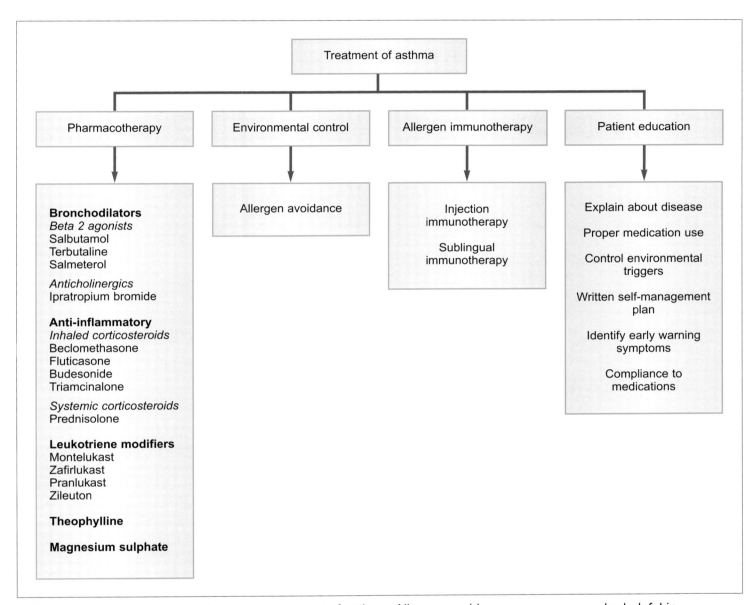

3.25 A comprehensive strategy for the management of asthma. Allergen avoidance measures may be helpful in reducing the severity of existing disease. Threshold concentrations of allergens that can be regarded as risk factors for acute attacks include: 10 μg/g dust of group 1 mite allergen; 8 μg/g dust of Fel d 1, the major cat allergen; 10 μg/g dust of Can f 1, the major dog allergen; and 8 μg/g dust of cockroach allergen. House dust mite avoidance is important for patients with house dust mite sensitivity. Removal of carpets and soft toys, and washing the bed linen at high temperatures are some of the methods employed for house dust mite avoidance.

Table 3.4 Classification of asthma severity by clinical features before treatment

Step 1: Intermittent
Symptoms less than once a week
Brief exacerbations
Nocturnal symptoms not more than twice a month
• FEV_1 or PEFR >80% predicted
• PEFR or FEV_1 variability <20%

Step 2: Mild persistent
Symptoms more than once a week, but less than once a day
Exacerbations may affect activity and sleep
Nocturnal symptoms more than twice a month
• FEV_1 or PEFR >80% predicted
• PEFR or FEV_1 variability 20–30%

Step 3: Moderate persistent
Symptoms daily
Exacerbations may affect activity and sleep
Nocturnal symptoms more than once a week
Daily use of inhaled short-acting β_2-agonist
• FEV_1 or PEFR 60–80% predicted
• PEFR or FEV_1 variability >30%

Step 4: Severe persistent
Symptoms daily
Frequent exacerbations
Frequent nocturnal asthma symptoms
Limitation of physical activities
• FEV_1 or PEFR <60% predicted
• PEFR or FEV_1 variability >30%

National Institutes of Health (2002). *Global Strategy for Asthma Management and Prevention*, pp. a1–a176

FEV_1, forced expiratory volume in 1 second; PEFR, peak expiratory flow rate

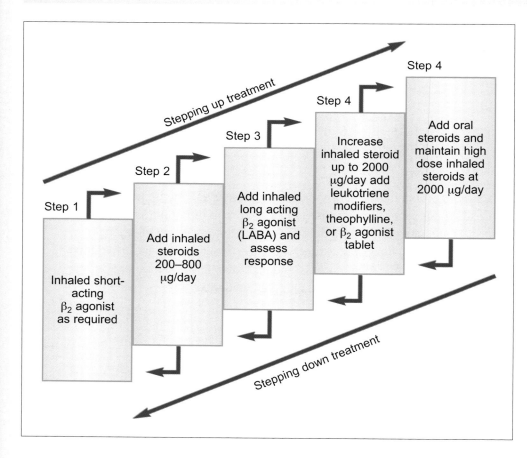

3.26 Stepwise management of asthma in adults. Some patients on long-acting beta agonist (LABA) may not show any response. In these individuals LABA may be stopped and the dose of inhaled steroids increased. If the response is poor, other groups of medications, such as leukotriene receptor antagonists or sustained release theophylline, can be considered. Step 1: Mild intermittent asthma. (Adapted from *Thorax* 2003; **58(Supplement I)**: 1–95.)

current treatment, and there is assurance the patient is using medication correctly (**3.26**). Inhaled steroids should be considered for patients with exacerbations of asthma in the last 2 years; using inhaled β_2 agonists three times a week or more and symptomatic three times a week or more, or for patients waking up due to symptoms.

Asthma exacerbations can be classified as mild, moderate, or severe. The presence of several, but not necessarily all factors indicate the severity of the asthma attack (*Table 3.1*, p46; **3.27**). Indicators of a life-threatening attack are: presence of bradycardia or hypotension; a silent chest with cyanosis; poor inspiratory effort; exhaustion,

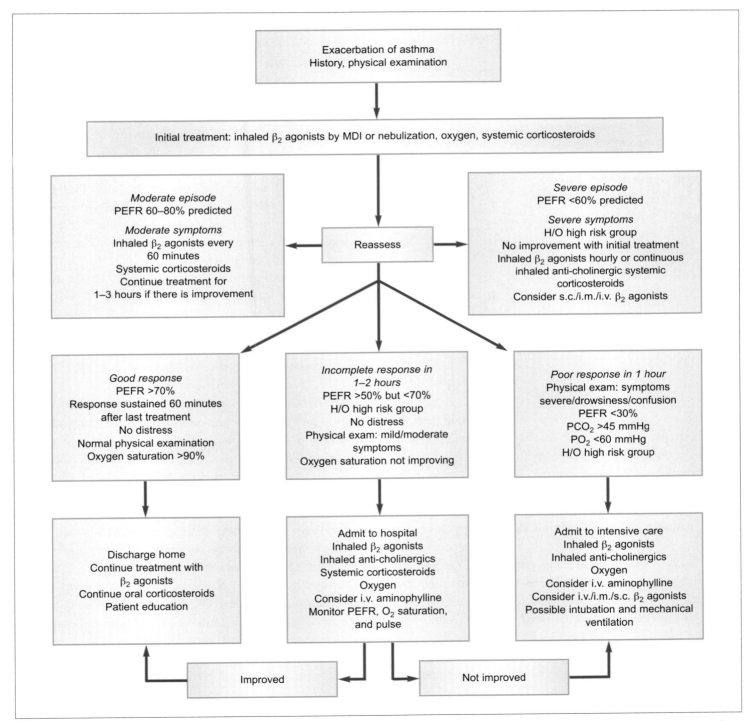

3.27 Approach to the management of acute severe asthma. (H/O, history of waking up due to symptoms; MDI, metered dose inhaler; PEFR, peak expiratory flow rate.)

Table 3.5 Risk factors associated with asthma deaths

- Past history of sudden severe exacerbation
- Prior intubation for asthma, or admission to intensive care
- Two or more hospitalizations for asthma in the past year
- Three or more visits to health centre for asthma in the past 4 weeks
- Use of two or more canisters of short-acting β_2 agonist in 1 month
- Current use or recent withdrawal of systemic corticosteroids
- Difficulty in perceiving airflow obstruction or its severity
- Co-morbidity from cardiovascular disease or chronic obstructive pulmonary disease
- Serious psychiatric illness
- Low socio-economic status
- Illicit drug use
- Sensitivity to alternaria

confusion, or coma; and a PEFR of <33%. Certain patients are at a higher risk of asthma-related deaths, and it is essential to do a risk factor assessment (*Table 3.5*). Patients with asthma exacerbation must follow an action plan provided to them by the health care provider. If they do not improve, admission to a hospital is indicated. An approach to the management of an asthma exacerbation is shown in **3.27**.

The prognosis for an asthma exacerbation is determined not by the presenting symptoms or by the severity of airflow obstruction, but by the response to treatment. In the majority of patients, symptoms resolve within 2 hours of initiating treatment. The principal goals of treatment of asthma exacerbations are correction of hypoxemia, reversal of airflow obstruction, and reduction of the likelihood of recurrences of airflow obstruction. The primary treatment for asthma includes oxygen, β_2 adrenoceptor agonists, and systemic corticosteroids.

Newer/experimental therapies for asthma

Corticosteroids have been the mainstay in the management of asthma, both in the acute scenario and in long-term management. Inhaled corticosteroids form the backbone of asthma therapy. However, corticosteroids are well known for their adverse effects on bone metabolism, suppression of the hypothalamopituitary axis (HPA) and other metabolic side-effects. Therefore, extensive research has been done in finding alternative anti-inflammatory therapies (**3.28**). The newer generation corticosteroids, such as ciclesonide, are metabolized locally, thus preventing the systemic absorption from the respiratory tract.

Theophylline, a non-selective phosphodiesterase (PDE) inhibitor, has been in use in the treatment of asthma for a long time. However, its narrow therapeutic window has precluded its routine use in patients with asthma. There are at least nine families of PDEs (PDE 1–9). PDE4 is of particular interest since it is thought to participate in regulating the function of a variety of inflammatory cells. Selective PDE4 inhibitors could be an answer to the side-effects seen with theophyllines.

Allergen immunotherapy is thought to act by up-regulating the Th1 and down-regulating the Th2 cytokine function. Various forms of allergen immunotherapy are being investigated as possible therapeutic approaches for asthma, such as allergen-derived peptide immunotherapy, immunostimulatory CpG oligonucleotides, DNA vaccines, and mycobacterial vaccination.

The advantage of the newer forms of immunotherapy (which include DNA and modified recombinant allergen vaccines) is that they have less local and systemic allergic reactions. This is due to the fact that these molecules have reduced or absent IgE binding, but at the same time they offer enhanced immunogenicity because of the large amount of immunogen that can be administered safely.

Cytokine modulation strategies essentially hinge on inhibition of pro-inflammatory cytokines, or augmenting the effects of anti-inflammatory cytokines. Certain cytokines have anti-inflammatory effects on allergic inflammation and, therefore, supplementing them has the potential to reduce airway inflammation. Inhibition of pro-inflammatory cytokines with blocking antibodies to cytokines, or their receptors, could also offer a novel therapeutic alternative.

The novel recombinant anti-IgE or omalizumab could be a useful adjunct in the treatment of asthma (**3.29**). It is a safe therapeutic modality, with an acceptable side-effect profile. Omalizumab reduces asthma exacerbations,

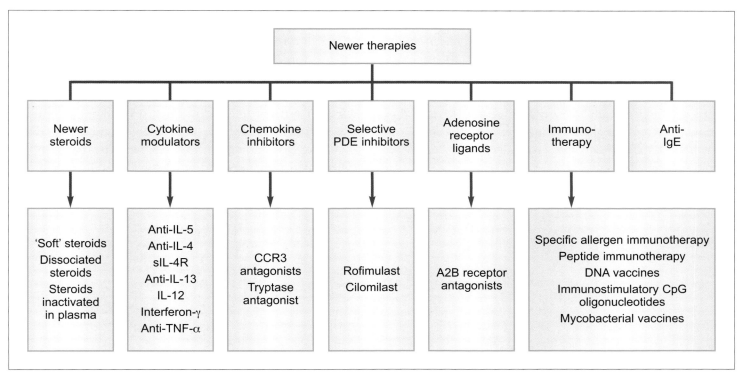

3.28 Newer and experimental therapies for asthma. (IL, interleukin; PDE, phosphodiesterase; TNF, tumour necrosis factor.)

3.29 Mechanism of action of anti-IgE. Of all the newer therapies being evaluated, blocking the effects of IgE at the high-affinity receptor site by a monoclonal anti-IgE antibody has shown promise, and is being approved for use in patients with asthma. Anti-IgE binds to free IgE and facilitates its removal, binds to membrane-bound IgE on B-cells, inhibiting IgE production by B-cells. However, it does not bind to IgE that is already bound to the IgE receptors on mast cells and basophils, because the epitope on IgE, against which they are directed, is already attached to those receptors, and hence, masked.

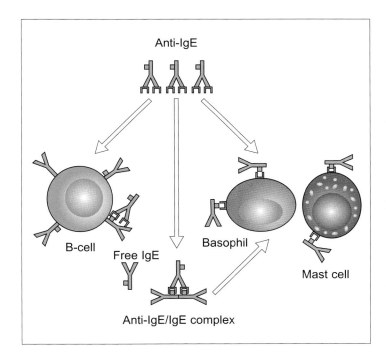

improves asthma symptom scores, improves lung function, improves quality of life and, most importantly, has a steroid sparing effect. The down regulation of the $Fc\varepsilon RI$ receptors on basophils by over 97% after treatment with omalizumab could further dampen the allergic cascade. The patient groups need to be defined clearly before embarking on this therapy. Severe asthmatics on very high doses of corticosteroids could find this especially useful due to its steroid sparing effects.

Despite all the advances in molecular biology, inhaled corticosteroids remain the anti-inflammatory therapy of choice in asthma, given the remarkable efficacy and overall safety. Targeting specific elements in the inflammatory cascade (such as IgE antagonists and cytokine modulators), may dampen the inflammatory cascade, but whether this is adequate remains to be seen. There are still unmet needs in the treatment of asthma, and future studies may give a better understanding of the relationships between the inflammatory changes and physiology, as well as the interactions with the currently available treatment modalities.

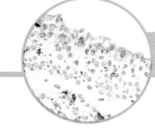

Chapter 4

Allergic rhinitis

Introduction

Rhinitis is defined as inflammation of the nasal membranes. It is characterized by a symptom complex that consists of any combination of the following: sneezing, nasal congestion, nasal itching, and rhinorrhea. Allergic rhinitis is one of the most common chronic conditions, and occurs in 15–20% of the population (**4.1**). The disease is uncommon under the age of 5 years. Most patients with allergic rhinitis develop symptoms before the age of 20 years. Allergic rhinitis usually improves in mid-life, and is seldom a problem in the elderly. A family history of allergic rhinitis and atopy increases the risk of a child developing the disease. While allergic rhinitis is not a life-threatening condition, complications can occur and the condition can significantly impair quality of life, which leads to a number of indirect costs. The total direct and indirect costs of allergic rhinitis were recently estimated to be $5.3 billion per year.

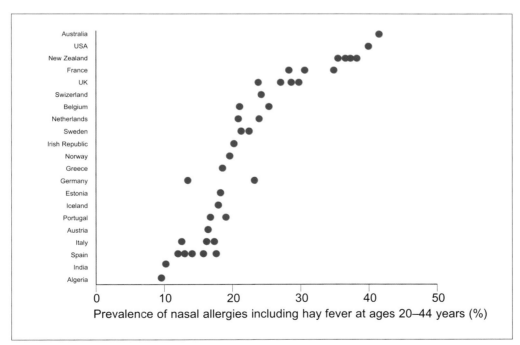

4.1 Establishing a reliable estimate of the prevalence of allergic rhinitis is difficult: prevalence estimates range from as low as 4%, to >40%. Epidemiology studies suggest the prevalence of allergic rhinitis is increasing in the US and around the world. The cause of this increase is unknown; however, contributing factors may include: higher concentrations of airborne pollution; rising dust mite populations; less ventilation in homes and offices; dietary factors; and the trend toward more sedentary lifestyles.

Pathophysiology

During the initial stage of the disease, low-dose allergen exposure leads to the production of specific IgE antibodies, which allows sensitivity to become established. A subsequent exposure to the allergen will trigger the allergic response. This IgE-mediated response is correlated with the clinical presentation of sensitization, acute-phase mast cell activation, acute-phase neuronal response, and the late-phase response. The early response is characterized by tingling and pruritus, sneezing, rhinorrhea, nasal congestion, and increased nasal resistance. Levels of exhaled NO are also increased.

Within 4–8 hours of allergen exposure, these cells release inflammatory mediators that bring about the late-phase response (**4.2**). The action of eosinophil-derived mediators leads to the clinical and histological appearance of chronic allergic disease. The repeated intra-nasal exposure to allergens then causes a brisk response to a reduced provocation. The release of Th2 cytokines in the nasal mucosa, with circulation to the hypothalamus, may give rise to systemic manifestations. Mast cell mediators promote the expression of vascular cell adhesion molecules and E-selectin, thus facilitating the adhesion of circulating leukocytes (such as basophils and eosinophils), to the endothelial cells, creating the cellular infiltrate characteristic of allergic rhinitis (**4.3, 4.4**).

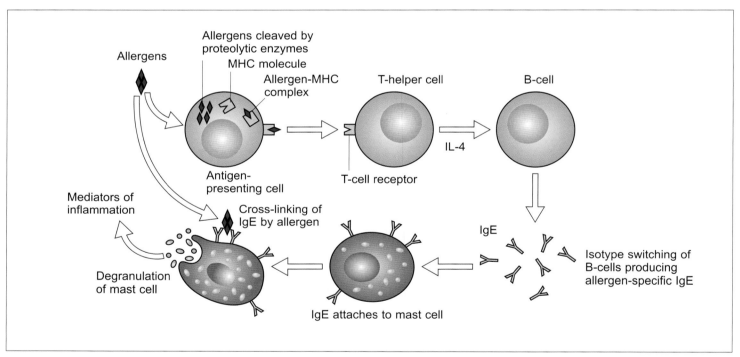

4.2 The mechanisms of allergic rhinitis involve both early- and late-phase responses. The early-phase response is attributed to IgE antibodies bound to tissue mast cells, which, upon exposure to an allergen, trigger an immediate release and formation of chemical mediators. Histamine, leukotrienes, bradykinin, and other chemical mediators are involved in this early-phase response. The immune response in allergy begins with sensitization. The antigen-presenting cells (such as Langerhans cells in the epithelium lining the airways of the lungs and nose), internalize, process, and then express these allergens on their cell surface. The allergens are then presented to other cells involved in the immune response, in particular, T-lymphocytes. Through a series of specific cell interactions, B-lymphocytes are transformed into antibody secretory cells – plasma cells. In the allergic response, the plasma cell produces IgE antibodies. The late-phase response results in priming and airway hyper-responsiveness. Priming is where up-regulation occurs in an area of inflammation and, upon secondary exposure to allergen, results in a heightened response to that allergen. (MHC, major histocompatibility complex.)

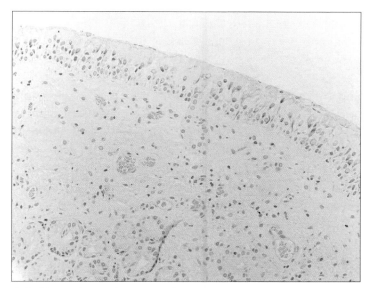

4.3 Normal nasal mucosa in a non-allergic subject showing no mast cells in the submucosa. (Courtesy of Mr R Salib, Southampton University.)

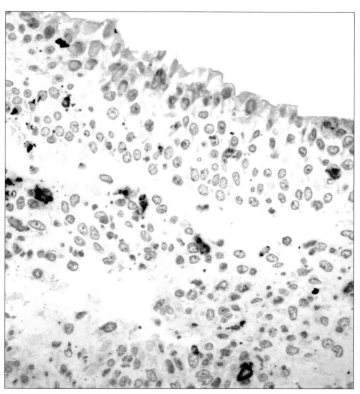

4.4 Immunohistochemical staining of nasal biopsies with monoclonal antibodies directed against mast cell tryptase shows an abundance of mast cells within the airway epithelium in both intermittent and persistent allergic rhinitis. (Courtesy of Mr R Salib, Southampton University.)

Diagnosis

The diagnosis of allergic rhinitis is dependent upon a thorough history and clinical examination (**4.5**). Laboratory tests are often required to strengthen the clinical diagnosis and to provide a means of objectively evaluating the disease, the degree of severity, and the efficacy of treatment (**4.6**). The most common tests employed in the diagnosis of

4.5 Diagnostic evaluation of allergic rhinitis.

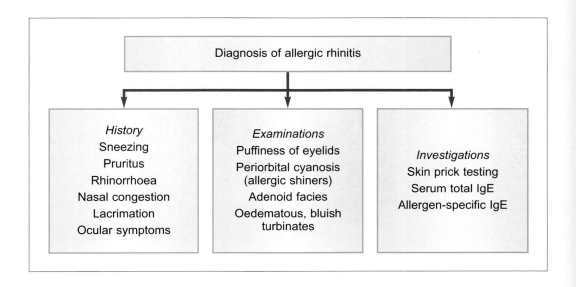

Diagnosis of allergic rhinitis

History
Sneezing
Pruritus
Rhinorrhoea
Nasal congestion
Lacrimation
Ocular symptoms

Examinations
Puffiness of eyelids
Periorbital cyanosis (allergic shiners)
Adenoid facies
Oedematous, bluish turbinates

Investigations
Skin prick testing
Serum total IgE
Allergen-specific IgE

allergic rhinitis are allergen-specific IgE levels and skin prick tests (SPTs). The clinical history should guide the clinician to test for the most relevant panel of allergens. It is important to note that a positive RAST or SPT, in the absence of a clear history, does not support the diagnosis of allergic rhinitis. Nasal biopsy and nasal lavage are research procedures and are rarely used in clinical practice (**4.7, 4.8**).

Allergic rhinitis can be classified as seasonal, perennial, or episodic (*Table 4.1*). Seasonal allergic rhinitis (SAR) is defined as: symptoms occurring during exposure to seasonal allergens, i.e. pollens of grasses, trees, and weeds (**4.9,**

4.10). Perennial allergic rhinitis (PAR) is defined as: nasal symptoms for more than 2 hours a day, for more than 9 months of the year. This happens when the patient is allergic to house dust mites, indoor moulds, animal danders, and cockroaches, or when patients are allergic to multiple seasonal allergens (**4.11**). Episodic allergic rhinitis refers to symptoms on exposure to allergens that are not normally in their environment, i.e. cat-allergic patients developing symptoms upon entering a house where there are cats. The severity of allergic rhinitis should also be assessed in accordance with recent guidelines (**4.12**).

Full blood counts, eosinophil count
SPT
Serum total IgE
RAST

X-ray sinuses to rule out sinusitis
CT scan sinuses
Nasal smears usually show eosinophilia
Rhinoscopy for evaluating structural abnormalities
Nasal provocation testing

4.6 Top panel: skin prick test (SPT) should be considered to elucidate the specific cause. Bottom panel: investigations are used in special situations to rule out other associated conditions. (CT, computed tomography; RAST, radio allergen sorbent test.)

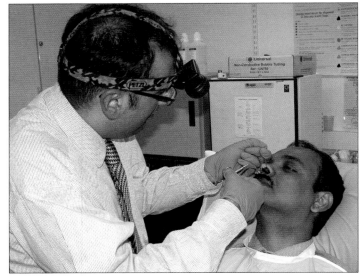

4.7 A nasal mucosal biopsy is usually used for research purposes to study the pathophysiological mechanisms of allergic rhinitis and the effects of treatment on the nasal mucosa.

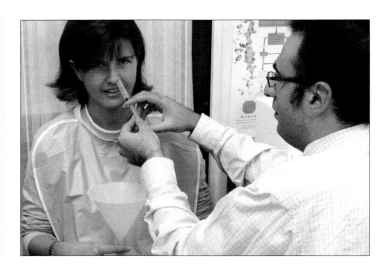

4.8 Nasal lavage is useful in evaluating the cellular population in allergic rhinitis. The anterior nares are lavaged by refluxing buffered saline, warmed to 37°C, with a syringe catheter apparatus. Nasal cytological examination is useful for the diagnosis of non-allergic rhinitis with eosinophilia syndrome (NARES). Intracellular bacteria and polymorphonuclear leukocytes are suggestive of an infectious process.

4.9 Pollen is a fine powder consisting of microgametophytes (pollen grains), which carry the male gametes of higher plants. Each pollen grain contains one or two generative cells (the male gametes) and a vegetative cell. Pollens that cause allergies are those of anemophilous (literally 'wind loving') plants, which produce very lightweight pollen grains in great quantities for wind dispersal, and subsequently come into contact with human nasal passages through breathing. Anemophilous plants generally have inconspicuous flowers.

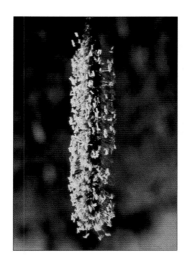

4.10 Ragweed, a yellow flowering weed, is a member of the aster family that often flourishes in disturbed vacant soils which cannot support other vegetation. It flourishes during dry, hot spells which promote growth and pollen formation. If these conditions continue through late summer, then pollen dispersal is very high. The only deterrent to making it difficult for the plant to release its pollen is relative humidity that exceeds 70%. One ragweed plant is capable of producing over a billion grains of pollen per season. There are some cross-reactivities exhibited by ragweed-allergic subjects. The cross-reactive allergens linked to ragweed include honeydew, cantaloupe, watermelon, banana, and chamomile. Avoidance of these foods is usually recommended to reduce compounding symptoms. A cross-reaction to ragweed pollen may cause oral allergy syndrome, which is itching or swelling of the lips, tongue, throat, or roof of the mouth.

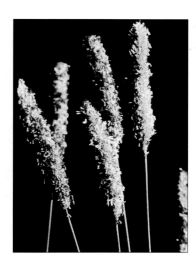

Table 4.1 Classification and differential diagnosis of allergic rhinitis

Allergic rhinitis	*Seasonal, perennial, episodic*
Non-allergic rhinitis	Vasomotor rhinitis – clear rhinorrhea, nasal congestion without exposure to allergens Cold air induced NARES – usually seen in adults, negative test for allergens and eosinophilia on nasal smears
Infectious rhinitis	Bacterial, fungal, and viral
Drug-induced rhinitis	Reserpine, OCP, rhinitis medicamentosa, beta blockers, hydralazine
Granulomatous rhinitis	Wegener's granulomatosis, sarcoidosis
Mechanical obstruction	Foreign body, deviated septum, adenoids
Tumours	Benign, malignant

NARES, non-allergic rhinitis with eosinophilia; OCP, oral contraceptive pill

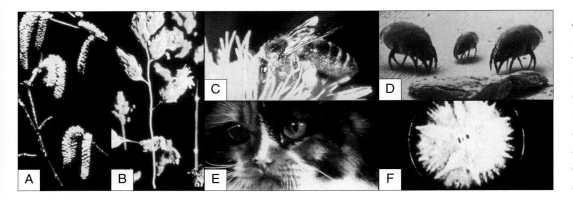

4.11 Seasonal allergic rhinitis, while called 'hay fever', is actually caused by airborne pollens from grasses and trees (**A–C**). House dust mites (**D**), animal dander (**E**), mould spores (**F**), and feathers commonly cause perennial allergic rhinitis. House dust mites are nearly universal in occurrence; a typical bed mattress may contain anything from 100,000 to 10 million mites. Ten per cent of the weight of a 2-year-old pillow may be composed of dead mites and their droppings. House dust mites are 0.2–0.3 mm long and translucent. Because of this, they are essentially invisible to the unaided eye. The most common species of dust mites are: the European house dust mite, *Dermatophagoides pteronyssinus* from the family Pyroglyphidae; and the North American house dust mite, *Der. farinae*. Patients become allergic to the proteins in the mite faecal pellets. The examination of house dust mite extracts has indicated that over 30 different proteins can induce IgE antibody production in patients allergic to the house dust mite. There are, however, dominant specificities, especially the group 1 and 2 allergens, which can account for much of the allergenicity of extracts. Of the 19 denominated allergens, major IgE binding has been reported for group 1, 2, 3, 9, 11, 14, and 15 allergens. However, other causes can include perfumes, chemicals, cigarette smoke, cleansers, and cosmetics. The specific offenders vary by season. Weeds are usually a problem from late summer to the first hard frost, grasses usually pollinate in the late spring and early summer, while trees pollinate in the spring, and outdoor moulds are largely a late winter/early spring problem.

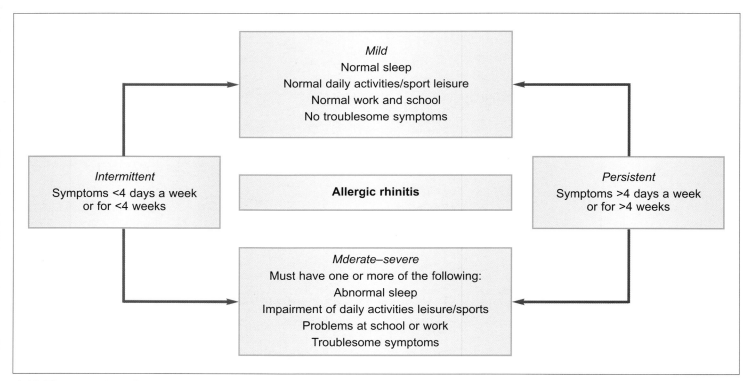

4.12 The new classification of allergic rhinitis (based on the allergic rhinitis and its impact on asthma [ARIA] guidelines) subdivides allergic rhinitis, in relation to the duration of the disease, into 'intermittent' or 'persistent' disease. The severity of allergic rhinitis is also classified as 'mild' or 'moderate–severe'. (Adapted from Bousquet J *et al.* [2001]. *J Allergy Clin Immunol*, **108**:s147–334.)

Physical examination helps to confirm the diagnosis, identify complications, and exclude other diagnoses (**4.13**). Long-standing obstruction due to adenoids leads to adenoid facies characterized by elongated face, open mouth, flattened malar eminences, pinched nostrils, raised upper lips, high-arch palate, and retracted jaws. In allergic rhinitis, the mucosa is pale and turbinates are hypertrophied (**4.14**). Nasal speculum examination might reveal purulent exudates and septal deviations. Anterior rhinoscopy is useful in ruling out co-existent nasal polyps and choanal atresia. Sinusitis may occur with long-standing disease and, rarely, infection may spread to the surrounding tissues (**4.15**).

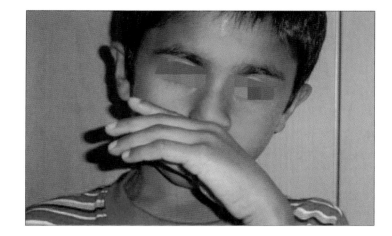

4.13 The allergic 'salute' refers to habitual rubbing of the nose due to constant irritation. It usually signifies an underlying allergic phenomena that is producing a profuse rhinorrhoea requiring frequent wiping. It is most marked in children.

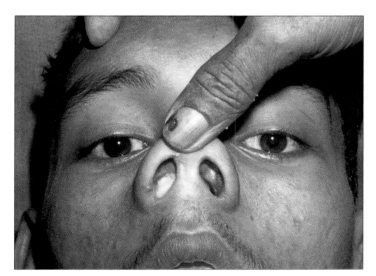

4.14 Patient with chronic perennial allergic rhinitis. The nasal mucosa is pale and both turbinates are hypertrophied. (Courtesy of Dr SH Abid, Dow Medical University, Karachi, Pakistan.)

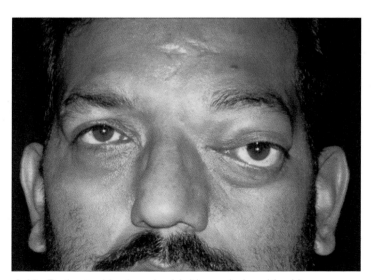

4.15 Patient with chronic rhinitis and sinusitis. He presented with swelling of the lateral aspect of the nose and left-sided proptosis. Investigations revealed allergic fungal sinusitis involving nose and left paranasal sinuses. (Courtesy of Dr SH Abid, Dow Medical University, Karachi, Pakistan).

Treatment of allergic rhinitis

Pharmacological treatment of allergic rhinitis should take into account these primary considerations: the efficacy, safety, and cost-effectiveness of medications; the patient's preference; and the objective of treatment. Since the progression and severity of allergic rhinitis are both correlated with environmental concentrations of the allergen causing the disease, allergen avoidance should be the first approach in the treatment of allergic rhinitis (**4.16**).

Pharmacological measures for the treatment of allergic rhinitis include antihistamines, corticosteroids, cromones,

Table 4.2 Therapeutic options in allergic rhinitis

Group	Examples	Remarks
First generation anti-histamines	Diphenhydramine Chlorpheniramine Hydroxyzine	Significant antimuscarinic effects, potent sedative, antimotion sickness Moderate sedation and antimuscarinic effects Low sedation, mainly used for motion sickness
First generation anti-histamines	Fexofenadine Azelastine Cetirizine Loratadine	No sedation Available as a nasal spray Occasional sedation reported
Topical corticosteroids	Beclomethasone Triamcinalone Flunisolide Mometasone Budesonide Fluticasone	Flurocarbon aerosol
Decongestants	Pseudoephedrine Phenylpropanolamine Phenylephrine	Rapid onset of action and continued usage can lead to rhinitis medicamentosa.
Cromones	Sodium cromoglycate	Used topically, safe in children and in pregnancy
Antileukotrienes	Montelukast Zileuton	Useful in patients not tolerating topical corticosteroids
Anticholinergics	Ipratropium bromide	Used in individuals in whom rhinorrhea is the predominant symptom

Antihistamines are the mainstay of therapy, but are not effective in controlling nasal congestion. Topical corticosteroids are the most effective treatment in allergic rhinitis, and can be used as the first line of therapy. Antileukotrienes are only useful in mild disease, and their efficacy can be enhanced when used in combination with antihistamines antileukotrienes, and decongestants (*Table 4.2*). Medications used for rhinitis are most commonly administered intra-nasally or orally.

The ARIA (Allergic Rhinitis and its Impact on Asthma) workshop report has suggested a step-wise treatment of allergic rhinitis (**4.17**). Allergen immunotherapy is effective in the treatment of allergic rhinitis and benefits may persist for several years after treatment has stopped (*Table 4.3*). It can modify the progression of allergic disease and may prevent the development of new allergies. Newer routes of administration are currently being investigated, such as sublingual immunotherapy and the use of purified allergens, T-cell reactive peptides, humanized anti-IgE monoclonal antibodies, and plasmid DNA immunization.

Table 4.3 A sample immunotherapy schedule

Dilution	Concentration	Volume (ml)	Dosage (SQ-U)
1:1000	100 SQ-U/ml	0.2	20
		0.4	40
		0.8	80
1:100	1000 SQ-U/ml	0.2	200
		0.4	400
		0.8	800
1:10	10,000 SQ-U/ml	0.2	2000
		0.4	4000
		0.8	8000
1:1	100,000 SQ-U/ml	0.1	10,000
		0.2	20,000
		0.4	40,000
		0.6	60,000
		0.8	80,000
		1.0	100,000

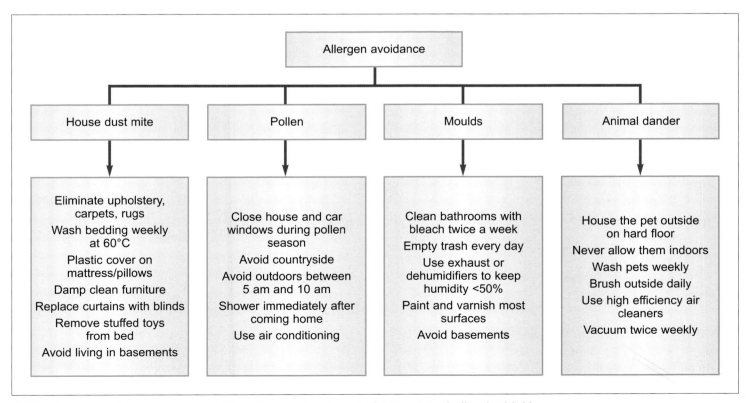

4.16 Allergen avoidance is essential for effective treatment of asthma and allergic rhinitis.

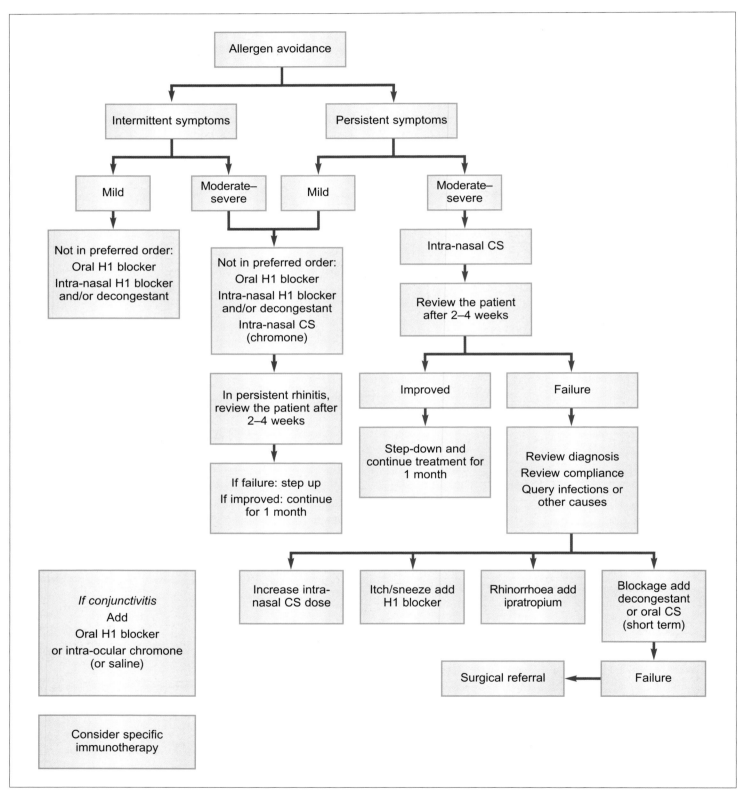

4.17 ARIA guidelines on the step-wise approach to the treatment of allergic rhinitis. (CS, corticosteroids.) (Adapted from Bachert C *et al.* [2002]. Allergic rhinitis and its impact on asthma. In collaboration with the World Health Organization. Executive summary of the workshop report. 7–10 December 1999, Geneva, Switzerland. *Allergy*, **57(9)**:841–55.)

Chapter 5

Atopic dermatitis

Introduction

Atopic dermatitis (AD) is part of the allergic diathesis. AD is a chronic inflammatory skin condition that affects 10–20% of children (**5.1**). The prevalence in adults is less certain but is reported to be <5% (**5.2**). AD is extremely common in infants and young children, but the vast majority grows out of it by the age of 5 years. New onset of AD after 5 years is uncommon

Pathogenesis

The pathogenesis of atopic dermatitis is complex with interplay of genetic and environmental factors (**5.3**). The skin of patients with AD is abnormally dry and irritable (dermal hyper-reactivity). Reduced skin barrier function due to loss of vital lipids leads to enhanced water loss and dry skin. These abnormalities can be demonstrated even in the uninvolved skin, and is largely genetically determined. Further genetic influence dictates the development of Th2 immune responses and inflammation (**5.4**). Environmental influences in the form of exposure to allergens, irritants, and infection contribute to the disease process.

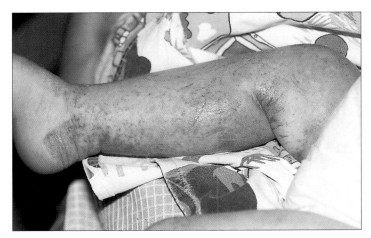

5.1 A young patient with AD.

5.2 Patient with extensive AD affecting most areas of the body including face and scalp. The skin is extremely dry and scaly with papules that are oozing, crusted, or excoriated.

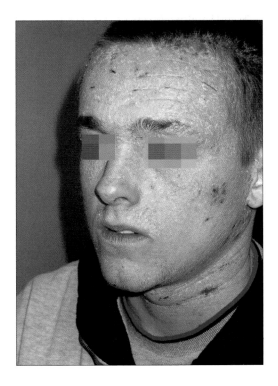

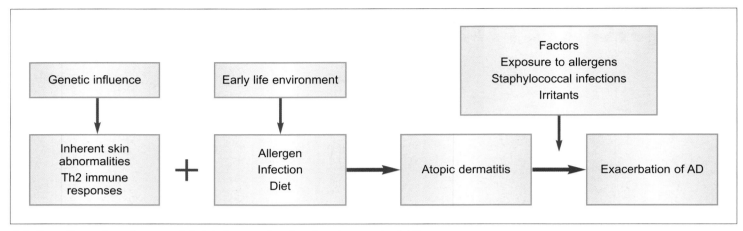

5.3 Genetic and environmental risk factors for the development of AD.

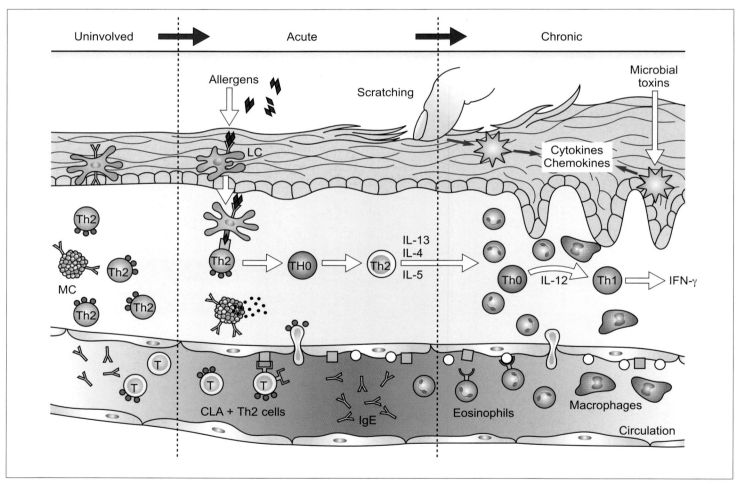

5.4 Evidence of Th2 immune response is present even in the uninvolved skin with the presence of T-lymphocytes (T) and IgE bearing Langerhans cells (LC) and mast cells (MC). This results in high serum IgE levels. Once the skin barrier is broken (scratching, inflammation), the allergen enters the skin to activate keratinocytes with the release of pro-inflammatory cytokines. These, in turn, cause an influx of inflammatory cells and the release of toxic mediators. Allergen sensitization occurs and Th2 type inflammation dominates the acute lesions. However, in chronic lesions, IL-12 production results in Th1 type inflammation with the production of interferon-gamma (IFN-γ). With superadded infection, bacterial antigens enhance the inflammatory process. (CLA, cutaneous lymphocyte-associated antigen; Th0, T-helper 0 cell.) (Modified from Leung DY [2000]. Atopic dermatitis: new insights and opportunities for therapeutic intervention. *J. Allergy Clin Immunol*, **105(5)**:860–76.)

Clinical features

The appearance varies depending on the age of the patient, chronicity of the lesions, and the effect of scratching and infection. In young children, the appearances are those of acute lesions that are intensely pruritic, erythematous papules, and vesicles with associated serous exudation (**5.5**). Histologically, these lesions demonstrate spongiosis. At this age, extensor surfaces are usually affected although, in more severe cases, any area of skin may be involved. In older children and adults, the lesions have a more chronic appearance with papules and excoriation on a hyper-pigmented and lichenified background (**5.6, 5.7**). The characteristic distribution involves flexural folds but hand and/or foot eczema may be the primary or sole manifestation in many adults. Various allergenic and irritant factors may exacerbate AD (*Table 5.1*).

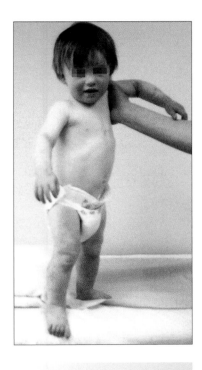

5.5 A young patient with AD showing extensive involvement of the face and extremities with acute erythematous lesions in a characteristic distribution.

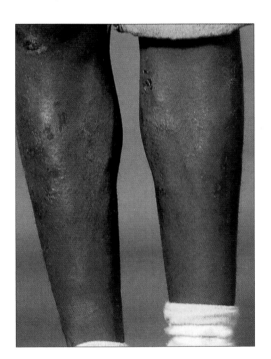

Table 5.1 Factors that may exacerbate symptoms in AD

- Temperature
- Humidity
- Irritants
- Infections
- Food allergen
- Inhalant allergen
- Contact allergens
- Emotional stress

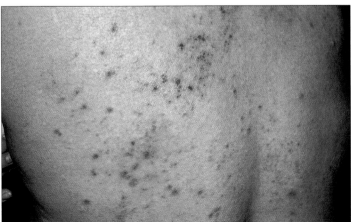

5.6, 5.7 AD in an older child (**5.6**) and adult (**5.7**) showing paulovesiuclar lesions on a thickened epidermis, which is hyper-pigmented. Signs of excoriation are visible.

Diagnosis

There are no objective tests and the diagnosis is based on clinical features (*Table 5.2*). To improve diagnostic accuracy, several diagnostic criteria, such as Hanifin and Rajkas, and UK working party criteria have been proposed. AD can mimic a number of other skin conditions (*Table 5.3*). The diagnosis should be revised if there is poor response to treatment. A skin biopsy may be needed in difficult cases.

Assessment of severity

The overall severity depends on the extent of skin involvement, the activity of AD lesions (assessed by erythema, excoriation, lichenification, oozing, and crusting),

the presence of infection, and response to treatment. SCORAD is an index, developed by the European Task Force on Atopic Dermatitis, for quantitative assessment of severity of AD. The SCORAD evaluates (1) the extent of the total body surface area that is affected; (2) the intensity of the condition based on six clinical features; and (3) subjective symptoms (**5.8**). The SCORAD Index assists the clinician in measuring and documenting the extent and severity of a patient's condition and response to treatment.

Management

Management of AD consists of avoidance of allergen/irritants, hydration of skin, suppression of inflammation, and treatment of complications, such as infection (**5.9**).

Table 5.2 Clinical features of AD

Mandatory	Morphology	Pruritic dermatitis with erythematous (acute), papular, and vesicular lesions
Typical	Course	Chronic or relapsing dermatitis
	Distribution	Face, neck, and extensor surfaces in infants and young children and flexural folds in older children and adults
Usual	Atopy	Personal and family history of atopic disease High total IgE Positive skin prick tests to common allergens
	Age of onset	Before 5 years
	Skin	Dryness, icthyosis Non-specific hand, foot, or scalp dermatitis
	Eye	Vernal conjunctivitis and keratoconus, cataract

Table 5.3 Differential diagnosis of AD

Chronic dermatoses	Seborrhoeic and contact dermatitis, nummular eczema, psoriasis, ichthyoses, lichen simplex chronicus, urticaria, and photosensitivity rash
Infections and infestations	Scabies, dermophytosis
Malignancies	Cutaneous T-cell lymphoma
Immunological disorders	Dermatitis herpetiformis, dermatomyositis
Immunodeficiencies	Wiskott–Aldrich, severe combined immunodeficiency disease, hyper-IgE, and DiGeorge syndrome
Metabolic disorders	Zinc, pyridoxine, or niacin deficiency and phenylketonuria

5.8 Calculation of SCORAD index for severity of AD: the area of involvement is calculated by adding all the areas involved, according to the rule of 9 (**A**). There are six severity criteria, graded on examination from 0–3 (0 = absence, 1 = mild, 2 = moderate, 3 = severe) and the total score added (**B**). Two subjective symptoms are graded on a scale of 0–10, and the score added (**C**). The scores of **A**, **B**, and **C** are put in the formula to get the SCORAD.

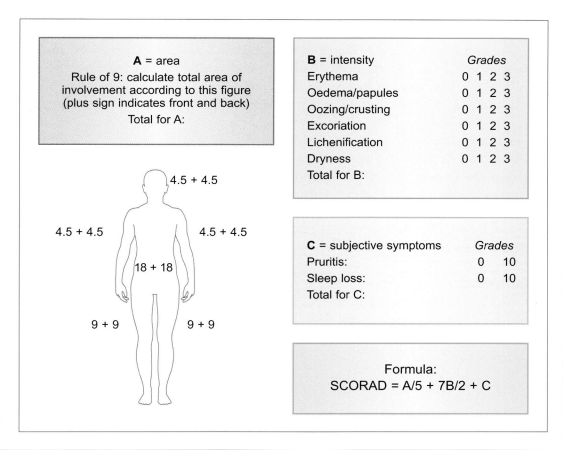

A = area
Rule of 9: calculate total area of involvement according to this figure (plus sign indicates front and back)
Total for A:

4.5 + 4.5

4.5 + 4.5   4.5 + 4.5

18 + 18

9 + 9   9 + 9

B = intensity	*Grades*
Erythema	0 1 2 3
Oedema/papules	0 1 2 3
Oozing/crusting	0 1 2 3
Excoriation	0 1 2 3
Lichenification	0 1 2 3
Dryness	0 1 2 3
Total for B:	

C = subjective symptoms	*Grades*
Pruritis:	0 10
Sleep loss:	0 10
Total for C:	

Formula:
SCORAD = A/5 + 7B/2 + C

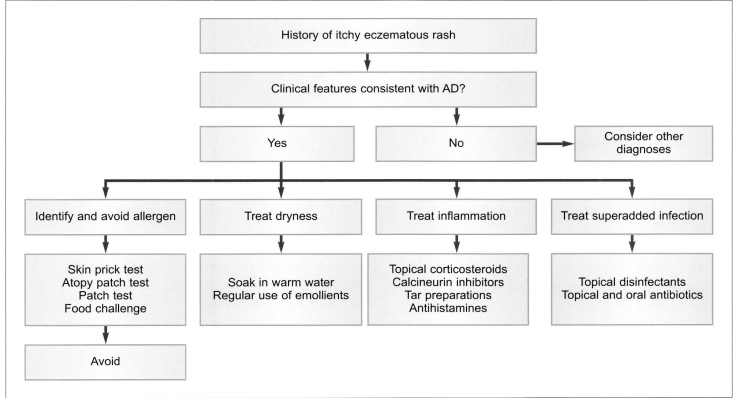

History of itchy eczematous rash

↓

Clinical features consistent with AD?

Yes → No → Consider other diagnoses

Identify and avoid allergen | Treat dryness | Treat inflammation | Treat superadded infection

Skin prick test
Atopy patch test
Patch test
Food challenge

Soak in warm water
Regular use of emollients

Topical corticosteroids
Calcineurin inhibitors
Tar preparations
Antihistamines

Topical disinfectants
Topical and oral antibiotics

Avoid

5.9 Initial management of AD.

Avoidance of allergen/irritants

Any relevant allergens should be identified using a skin test, or measurement of specific IgE in the blood. The relevance of a positive test should always be interpreted with information available from the history. Food challenge may be required to determine the relevance of a positive test. Patients with AD may develop contact sensitization, and a patch test may be needed if there is a suggestive history. Patient education is important with regard to avoidance of relevant allergens, as well as irritants, such as direct application of soaps, perfumes, and cosmetics. Advice regarding avoidance should be explained to the patient, and written information given for future reference (*Table 5.4*).

Skin hydration

AD patients should use Vaseline™ or ointment-based moisturizers, such as petroleum jelly or an emulsifying ointment. These are more effective than creams. Moisturizers should be applied several times a day and should be used on top of topical steroids.

Anti-inflammatory medication

Topical corticosteroids are the mainstay of treatment and should be applied to the involved skin (**5.10**). Appropriate potency should be used (*Table 5.5*). Corticosteroids should not be used regularly, on the same area of the skin for long periods in view of adverse effects, such as skin atrophy, striae, and folliculitis. Systemic absorption depends on the area applied, potency of the steroids, and use of occlusive dressing. Wet (occlusive) dressings prevent scratching, keep skin hydrated, and let topical steroids work on the skin for a longer period of time. They have been shown to be effective in more difficult cases of AD (**5.11**).

Calcineurin inhibitors, such as tacrolimus and pimecrolimus, have anti-inflammatory activity in terms of suppression of lymphocyte activation and inhibition of other inflammatory cells in AD. They reduce pruritis, improve condition of AD lesions and, following long-term use, reduce the number of exacerbations and requirement of topical steroids. They have been proven to be relatively safe and well tolerated. Cyclosporine is an effective, though

---

Table 5.4 Information and advice on skin care in AD

- Keep skin clean but avoid frequent washing
- Soak the area in warm water
- The skin should be patted dry, not rubbed
- Avoid direct contact with chemicals, such as soaps, detergents, cosmetics
- Avoid warm, occlusive clothing
- For clothing and bedding, avoid wool or synthetic material. A non-irritant material, such as cotton, is preferable
- Use moisturisers at least twice a day and after each wash
- Nails should be cut regularly to avoid scratching and infection. Infant's hands may need to be covered at night to prevent scratching
- There is no good evidence that ingestion of certain oils improve skin hydration
- Treat exacerbations and infections promptly

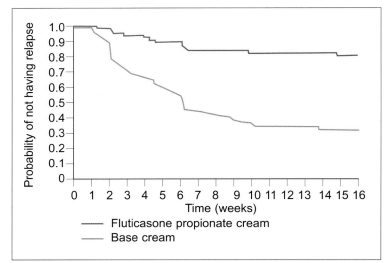

5.10 Topical corticosteroid are effective treatment for AD. This study shows that the risk of relapse reduced significantly following twice weekly maintenance treatment with topical corticosteroid. (Modified from Berth-Jones J *et al.* [2003]. Twice weekly fluticasone propionate added to emollient maintenance treatment to reduce risk of relapse in atopic dermatitis: randomised, double blind, parallel group study. *BMJ*, **326(7403)**:1367.)

Table 5.5 Use of appropriate potency of topical corticosteroids for AD

Potency	Examples	Indications
Mild	Hydrocortisone 1%	Mild AD
		Face, eyelids, intertriginous areas
		Infants
Moderate	Clobetasone butyrate 0.05%	Moderate disease
		During exacerbation
Potent	Betamethasone valerate 0.1%	Severe AD
		During flare-up of moderate to severe disease
Very potent	Clobetasol propionate 0.05%	For short period only, for disease not responding to less potent steroids

Lowest potency which is effective should be applied thinly, twice a day

potentially toxic treatment option for severe AD. It is usually given at 5 mg/kg/day, with careful monitoring of blood pressure and renal function.

Tar preparations are widely used in the treatment of AD, but evidence from randomized controlled trials is lacking. These should not be used on acutely inflamed skin. An antihistamine may reduce itching, but clear evidence of its antipruritic effect in AD is lacking. However, sedating antihistamines, such as chlorpheniramine, can have a beneficial effect in infants and children with sleep disturbance due to itching.

Infections

Staphylococcal infections are common and nearly always present in acute (wet) stages. For mild infection (**5.12**), topical antibiotics, such as bactroban, applied twice a day, may be sufficient. For extensive infectious eczema, skin cleansing with an antimicrobial, such as chlorhexadine, may be needed. It should be followed by a course of oral antibiotics, such as flucloxacillin or cephalosporins (**5.13**).

The response to therapy should be monitored and further action taken, as necessary (**5.14**). It is important to exclude allergens and irritants from the patient's environment before using potent steroids or other potentially toxic treatment. If the response to therapy remains inadequate, the diagnosis should be reviewed.

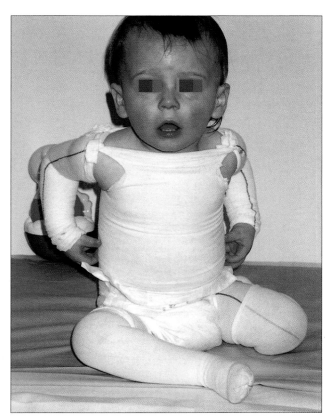

5.11 A patient with severe AD has had topical treatment of steroids and emollients under occlusive dressing for maximum effect.

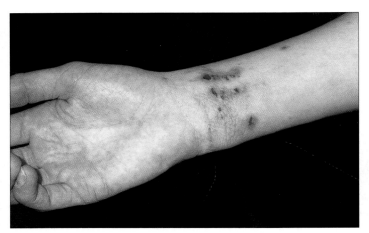

5.12 In chronic AD, scratching leads to bleeding, oozing, and infection.

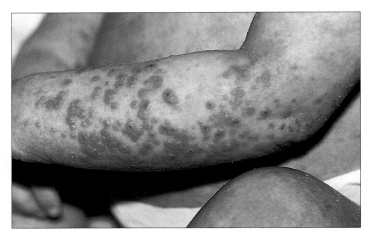

5.13 This severely infected AD improved following a course of systemic antibiotic.

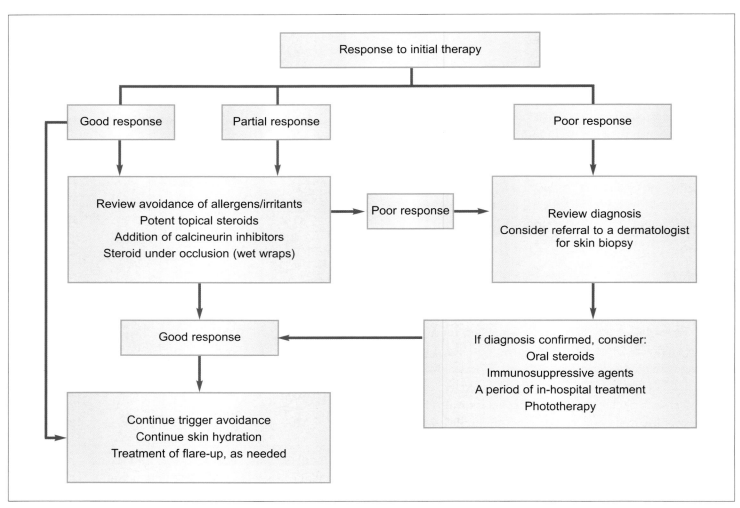

5.14 Follow-up management of AD.

Chapter 6

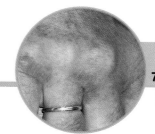

Contact dermatitis

Introduction

Contact dermatitis (CD) refers to adverse cutaneous reactions resulting from direct contact with an external agent. It is a common inflammatory skin condition that primarily affects older children and adults. CD can be allergic (ACD) or irritant (irritant CD). In some cases of ACD, exposure to sunlight is required for sensitization (photoallergic CD). CD is often due to a chemicals encountered at work (occupational CD), which may have serious financial implications.

Common sensitizing agents for ACD include nickel, plants (e.g. poison ivy), and occupational sensitizers (e.g. epoxy resins) (*Table 6.1*). Latex can cause immediate (IgE-

mediated) reactions, as well as ACD. A concurrent allergic or irritant CD may also develop from non-latex chemicals used in rubber. In irritant CD, skin irritants produce eczematous skin changes. In photoallergic CD, exposure to sun light (i.e. ultraviolet light) is essential for the initiation of an allergic response to the offending agent. Thus, it affects exposed areas, such as the face and arms. Work-related skin diseases account for approximately 50% of occupational illnesses (**6.1, 6.2**). Industries in which workers are at highest risk include manufacturing, food production, construction, printing, metal plating, leather work, and cosmetics.

Table 6.1 Common causes of ACD

Groups	Examples
Metals	Nickel sulphate, cobalt chloride
Cosmetics	Balsam of Peru, fragrance mix
Rubber products	Latex, thiuram mix, mercaptobenzothiazole, mercapto mix, black rubber mix, carba mix
Preservatives	Thimerosal, formaldehyde, quaternium-15, potassium dichromate, paraben mix, ethylenediamine dihydrochloride
Glues, plastic	Epoxy resin, *para*-tertiary-butylphenol formaldehyde resin, colophony
Dyes	*Para*-phenylenediamine
Antibiotics	Neomycin sulphate
Vehicle (creams, lotions)	Wool alcohol

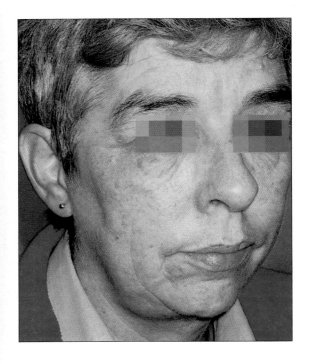

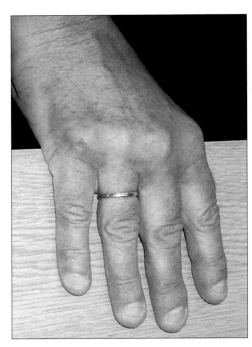

6.1, 6.2 This patient worked in a supermarket staff canteen. She had irritant CD of face and hands to the disinfectant spray she was using to clean the surfaces. Dryness and scaling on a background of erythema are main features of chronic irritant CD. The patch test was negative, but symptoms improved when the use of the disinfectant spray was stopped.

Pathophysiology

ACD results from an antigen-specific, lymphocyte-mediated hyper-sensitivity reaction. The effector cells are CD8 T-cells, whereas CD4 T-cells function as regulatory cells. Most antigens causing ACD are small molecules that may act as hapten, and bind to protein to form an antigen. These molecules are absorbed through the skin and activate epidermal Langerhans cells, which in turn stimulate naïve T-cells to generate antigen-reactive CD8 and CD4 cells (sensitization). Further exposure to the specific antigen leads to inflammatory cellular exudates and release of toxic mediators, with clinically evident ACD.

Irritant CD involves a non-immunologic response to a mild skin irritant, such as solvents or soaps. Prolonged exposure causes disturbance of cell hydration as a result of the defatting action of irritants, with resultant xerosis of the skin.

Clinical manifestations

CD is characterized by clearly demarcated areas of rash at sites of exposure. Acute lesions are pruritic vesicles on a background of erythema (**6.3**). In subacute stages, erythema and scaling are prominent, although some vesiculation may persist. Chronic lesions are characterized by dryness, lichenification, and scaling. The rash usually improves on removal of the offending agents but this is not always the case, especially if the exposure period has been long.

Appearances of different forms of CD are similar to each other and indeed may be indistinguishable from AD (*Table 6.2*). Other differential diagnoses include nummular eczema, seborrheic dermatitis, and psoriasiform dermatitis.

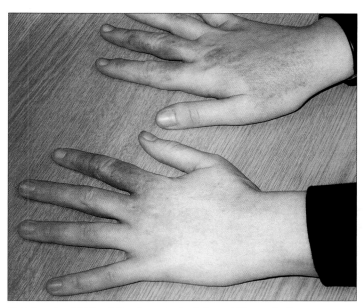

6.3 Acute ACD of the hands to latex. Although there was a positive reaction on skin prick test to latex, there was no clinical evidence of immediate reactivity to latex. The patient had a negative patch test to other rubber constituents on patch test, but had a positive challenge to rubber gloves ('glove finger test').

Table 6.2 Features differentiating AD and CD

	AD	*CD*
Distribution	Flexural folds	Hands, feet, face, eyelids, or site of contact
Family history of atopic disease	Commonly present	Commonly absent
Allergic asthma or allergic rhinitis	Commonly present	Commonly absent
Total IgE	High	Normal
Test	Positive skin prick tests	Positive patch test
Age of onset	<5 years	>5 years

Both diseases present with chronic or chronically relapsing erythematous and papulovesicular dermatitis

Management

Diagnosis

A detailed history, including occupational history, is mandatory. The appearance of CD may coincide with taking up of a new job or a new chemical process initiated at work, which may have led to exposure to a contact sensitizer (**6.4**). However, sometime patients present with chronic dermatitis with no clear history of exposure to a particular allergen or irritant.

CD initially involves the area of the skin that has been directly exposed but later it may spread to adjacent areas and more distant sites. The distribution of CD often provides support for the diagnosis and clues to the specific cause (*Table 6.3*). An erythematous scaling plaque in areas where metal jewelry is in contact with the skin is suggestive of ACD to nickel. Face and eyelids dermatitis is often due to a cosmetic allergy (**6.5**). Hands may be involved in ACD due to occupational exposure. ACD to plants is often characterized by linear lesions. Photoallergic dermatitis involves the more exposed areas of skin (face, hands, and feet). In contrast, textile-related allergens produce dermatitis of clothed areas. Poor response to standard treatments of AD should also suggest the possibility of ACD, as an alternative or concomitant diagnosis.

Patients should be patch tested when contact allergy is suspected. Patch testing is a procedure that is well-characterized, and the reactions are quantified with a validated scoring system (*Table 6.4*). The standard battery incorporates antigens that will cause most cases of ACD (70–80%). However, there are nearly 3,000 potential environmental allergens, and more extensive testing may be required. This might involve incorporation of additional chemicals into the patch testing procedure, depending on the history and the specific circumstances (**6.6**). Alternatively, offending agents may be tested under conditions of normal use (**6.7**). Interpretation of patch testing should always be done with clues obtained from the history and physical examination, as both false–positive and false–negative reactions occur. Photopatch testing may be useful when photoallergic dermatitis is suspected. In difficult cases, skin biopsy may be indicated to exclude other diagnoses, but it may not confirm CD.

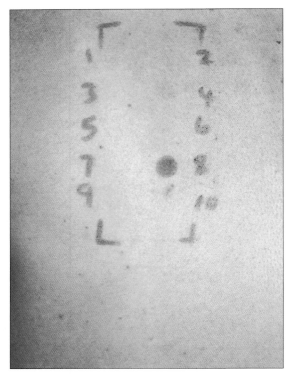

6.4 This patient developed ACD of hands and face 3 months after taking a factory job using glues to join fibreglass items. Patch test to a standard battery revealed a positive reaction to epoxy resin. He was moved to a different area of the factory which resulted in resolution of his symptoms.

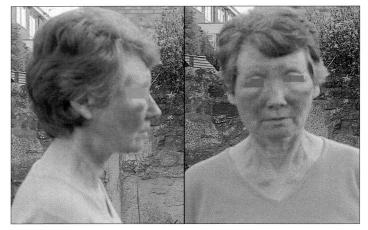

6.5 ACD of the face due to cosmetics.

Table 6.3 Causes of ACD according to the area affected

Area affected	Common causes
Eyelids	Cosmetics, poison ivy
Hands	Rubber products, epoxy resin, preservatives
Face	Cosmetics, UV light, wool alcohol, hair dyes
Neck	Nickel, cosmetics
Trunk	Nickel, rubber
Axilla	Deodorants, detergents, formaldehyde
Lower legs	Neomycin, epoxy resin

Table 6.4 American Contact Dermatitis Society patch test interpretation

Grade	Characteristics
+++	Coalescing vesiculobullous papules
++	Erythema, oedema, discrete vesicles
+	Erythema, infiltration, discrete papules
±/?	Doubtful reaction, macular erythema
-	No reaction
IR	Irritant response

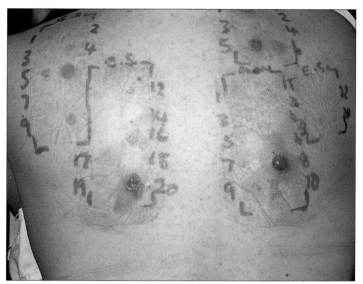

6.6 This patient worked as a beautician, dying eyelashes. She reacted on standard battery (applied on the left side) to fragrance mix (mild reaction) and p-phenylenediamine, present in hair dyes (strong reaction). In addition, she had moderate to strong reactions to the dyes she was using at work (patch test applied on the right side).

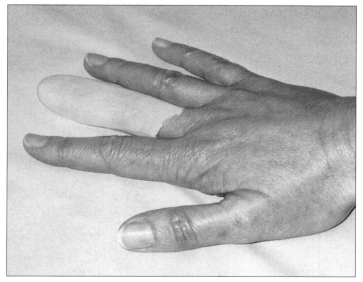

6.7 Latex glove finger test. A 'use test' may be helpful where there is a history of a dermal reaction on direct contact.

Treatment

Identification and removal of the offending agent is the mainstay of treatment of CD (**6.8**). The history might be suggestive of an allergen, but this should be confirmed with a patch test. Once identified, the allergen or irritant should be excluded from the patient's environment. However, this may not always be possible, especially for occupational agents. Gloves and protecting gear should be used by all workers exposed to known sensitizing agents, and may provide a solution for mild sensitizing agents for patients who are not able to change occupation. If the history does not provide a clue, patch test to a standard battery may be helpful, but any positive result should be interpreted with caution. If a patch test is negative, the diagnosis should be reviewed. If no agent can be found, symptomatic treatment may be the only option.

Barrier creams may help with dryness, and antihistamines might provide some relief from itching. Exacerbations should be treated with high-potency, topical corticosteroids and, occasionally, a course of oral steroid may be needed. Severe ACD may require phototherapy or other anti-inflammatory agents.

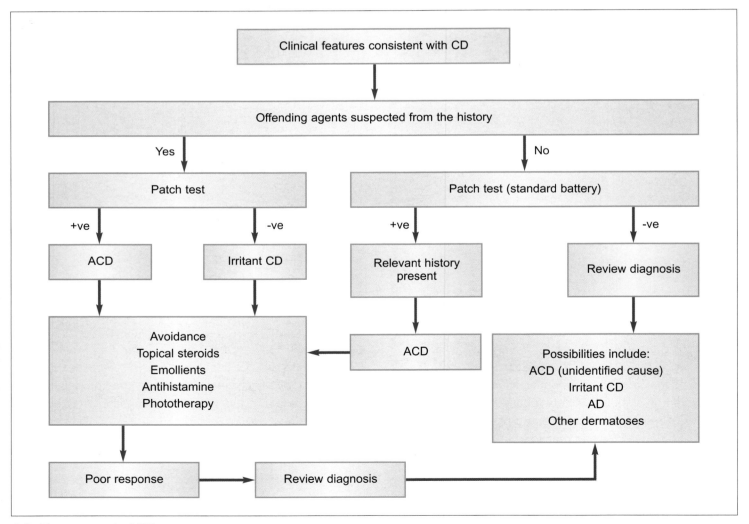

6.8 Management of CD.

Chapter 7

Urticaria and angioedema

Introduction

Urticaria is a localized, usually well-demarcated area of oedema within superficial layers of the skin (**7.1**). Angioedema occurs in the deeper layers of the skin and mucous membrane, and is less well demarcated. Urticarial lesions are erythemtous with a pale centre, ranging from 1–2 mm to several centimetres in diameter, and are often pruritic (**7.2**). Angioedema presents as diffuse swelling and may be painful (**7.3**). Urticaria and angioedema may occur in isolation (40% and 10%, respectively), or they may be present concomitantly (50%). In some cases, episodes last for more than 48 hours and leave a residual mark. In these cases, vasculitis or autoimmune mechanism should be suspected.

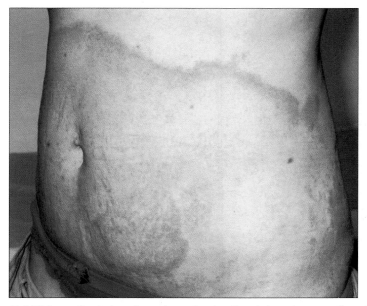

7.1 This patient developed marked urticarial rashes on the abdomen. Although she suspected foods, no cause could be found on investigation.

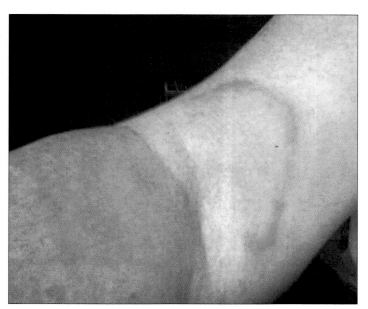

7.2 An example of an urticarial rash spanning several centimetres in diameter.

7.3 Angioedema affecting the right lower leg. Typical features of diffuse erythematous swelling can be clearly seen.

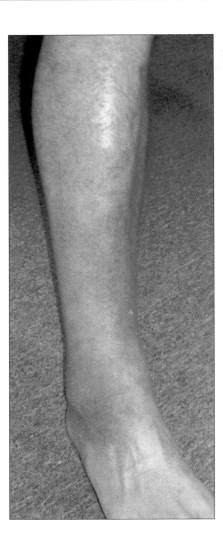

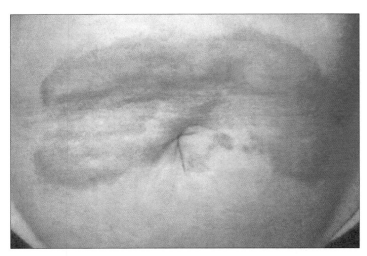

7.4 Generalized urticaria in a young patient. This was an acute, isolated episode and probably due to a viral infection.

Urticaria and angioedema are common diseases with an estimated prevalence of 0.5–1%, and approximately 15% of the population is affected at least once during their lifetime. It can occur at any age, but young adults are more frequently affected (**7.4**). It can be acute or chronic (repeated episodes for >6 weeks). In chronic urticaria, individual lesions are transient, usually persisting for <24 hours, but new lesions appear and disappear over a period of time (**7.5**). Chronic idiopathic urticaria runs a course of relapse and remissions over a period of years or decades. The duration of a relapse is difficult to predict in an individual and may vary from weeks to years. Hereditary angioedema is characterized by recurrent attacks (without urticaria). These involve skin and upper respiratory or GI tracts, with a duration of hours to days. Laryngeal oedema may be life threatening.

7.5 This patient had chronic recurrent urticaria with individual lesions lasting for 24–48 hours.

Pathogenesis

Mast cell degranulation in the skin (both IgE- and non-IgE-mediated) is the common underlying event. Many factors can trigger mast cell degranulation including food and food additives, drugs, and physical factors. Histamine is the most important mediator released by mast cells, and most of the features of urticaria and angioedema (tissue oedema, vascular dilatation, and itching) are due to histamine effects. Other mediators, such as LTs, PGs, platelet-activating factor, and TNF-α may also contribute to the pathogenesis. Histologically, there is oedema of the epidermis and dermis, with post-capillary venule leakage and, in later stages, infiltration of inflammatory cells.

Acute urticaria is often due to immediate (IgE-mediated) hyper-sensitivity as part of a systemic allergic reaction, and sometime urticaria and/or angioedema may be the sole manifestation (**7.6**). Immune complex mechanism is also implicated in acute urticaria (drugs, blood, and blood products). Chronic recurrent urticaria has a number of recognized triggers but in the majority (80–90%), none can be found (idiopathic urticaria). In 40% of these cases, autoantibodies of IgG class, directed against the α subunit of the high-affinity IgE receptor (FcϵR1α), can be shown to be present. These antibodies can induce histamine release from basophils and mast cells bearing FcϵR1 (**7.7**). The urticarial lesions tend to last longer than 24 hours in these patients. Heredity angioedema is due to a deficiency of C1 inhibitor (C1INH) levels, or its functional component. An acquired deficiency of C1INH may occur with lymphoproliferative disorders, or due to accelerated consumption of the enzyme by circulating autoantibodies.

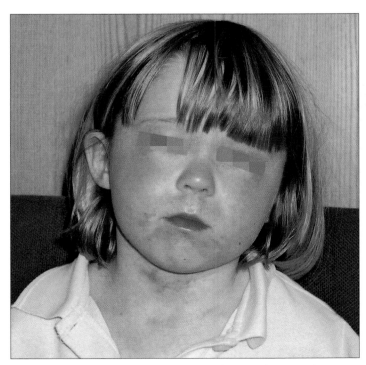

7.6 This patient had an acute allergic reaction to a horse with prominent angioedema of the face. Skin prick test confirmed a high sensitivity to horse allergen.

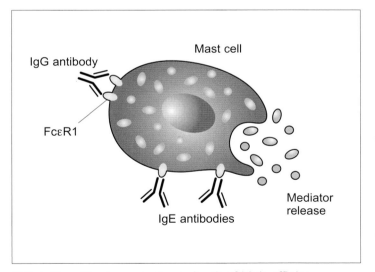

7.7 IgG antibody against α subunit of high affinity receptor, on the surface of mast cells, cross-link adjacent receptors to initiate degranulation and release of mediators.

Management

Diagnosis

Urticaria and angioedema are clinical diagnoses. If the lesions are present at the time of examination, it is relatively easy to establish the nature of the rash. Acute urticaria and angioedema can be quite dramatic with erythema and rash all over the body surface and swelling of the face, lips, and tongue (**7.8**). Angioedema should be differentiated from other causes of facial swelling (**7.9**). In chronic urticaria, a history of recurrent transient wheals of different sizes and shapes involving several areas of the skin is sufficient for the diagnosis, in most cases (**7.10, 7.11**).

The history should focus on possible triggering factors. In acute urticaria and angioedema, the attacks may be precipitated by known triggers (such as exposure to allergens) or may occur without any identifiable event. The causes are similar to those of systemic allergic reactions (*Table 7.1*). Hence, skin prick test or measurement of specific IgE might be helpful in elucidating or confirming an aetiology. If the history is suggestive of physical urticaria, the specific cause should be identified (*Table 7.2*). For example, application of an ice cube to the volar forearm for 5 minutes, with follow-up observation for 10–15 minutes, might confirm cold urticaria. In pressure urticaria, dermographism could usually be elicited. If an associated systemic disease is suspected, such as thyroid disease, appropriate test might be indicated for confirmation. C1INH levels should be checked if there is a family history or in those with severe angioedema. For drugs or food additives, a period of exclusion and challenge may be the only way to establish the cause.

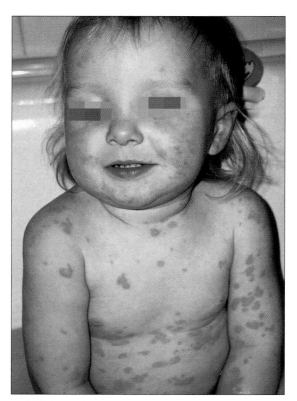

7.8 This patient had acute urticaria and angioedema, which was investigated and was found to be due to peanut allergy.

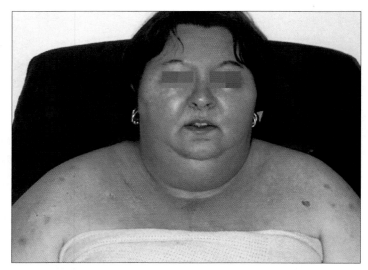

7.9 This patient presented to the allergy clinic with diffuse swelling of the face and neck and a provisional diagnosis of angioedema was made. However, further investigation revealed that she had obstruction of superior vena cava due to bronchogenic carcinoma (pancoast tumour).

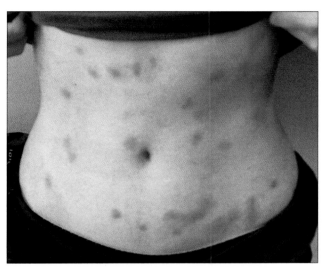 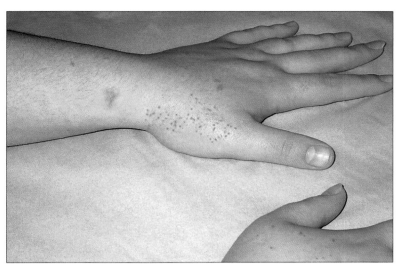

7.10, 7.11 Typical examples of urticarial rash on the trunk and arm.

Table 7.1 Common causes of urticaria and angioedema

Acute	Allergens	Foods: peanut, tree nuts, egg, cow's milk, fish, shellfish , fruits
		Inhalant: pollens (grass, ragweed), animal (cat, horse)
	Drugs	Aspirin, non-steroidal anti-inflammatory agents, angiotensin-converting enzyme inhibitors, radiocontrast media, progesterone
	Infections	Viral
	Other causes	Insect sting, allergen-specific immunotherapy, latex
Chronic	Physical	Heat, cold, water, sunlight, pressure, stress
	Autoimmune	Gastritis, systemic lupus erythematosus
	Infections	Sinusitis, parasitic infections, candidiasis
	C1 inhibitor deficiency	Hereditary, acquired
	Systemic diseases	Thyroid disease, masteocytosis
	Foods	Food additives, natural salicylate
	Idiopathic	–

Table 7.2 Types of physical urticaria

Type	Irritant
Pressure urticaria and dermographism	Pressure or minor trauma
Delayed-type pressure urticaria	Onset occurs 4–6 hours after pressure
Cold urticaria	Exposure to cold, usually confined to the exposed area
Cholinergic urticaria	Changes in core body temperature associated with exercise, hot showers and baths, fever, and anxiety
Exercise-induced urticaria	Vigorous physical exertion
Heat-induced urticaria	Exposure to heat, usually confined to area of exposure
Solar urticaria	Exposure to natural or artificial light
Aquagenic urticaria	Exposure to water

Treatment

Acute urticarial episode should be treated with antihistamine, but epinephrine may be needed, if life threatening features are also present (**7.12**). Once the cause is established, it should be completely avoided. If a systemic disease or chronic infection is uncovered, this should be treated appropriately. In physical urticaria, the triggering factor should be identified and avoided as much as possible. However, in many cases of physical and idiopathic urticaria and angioedema, the treatment relies on suppression of symptoms (**7.13**).

Antihistamines are the mainstay of treatment. Non-sedative antihistamines are preferred (cetirizine, fexofenadine, loratadine, and desloratadine), and these should be given on a regular basis in chronic recurrent urticaria. If the response is inadequate, the dose of antihistamine could be increased or a sedative antihistamine added at bed time.

A period of 3–6 months may be needed until remission is induced. In some patients with partial response to antihistamines, H_2 receptor antagonists and LT antagonists may be added. A severe episode may require a short course of oral steroid. Regular use of systemic corticosteroids or immunosuppressive treatments (e.g. cyclosporine) should be reserved for the most severe cases of urticaria, who are not responding to other treatment. For patients with severe urticaria, known to be due to anti-FcεR1 autoantibodies, plasmapheresis and intravenous gamma-globulin therapy have been used successfully. Treatment of acute exacerbation in C1INH deficiency includes intravenous purified C1INH concentrate. Prophylactic management in C1INH deficiency involves regular use of attenuated androgens, such as danazol or antifibrolytic drugs.

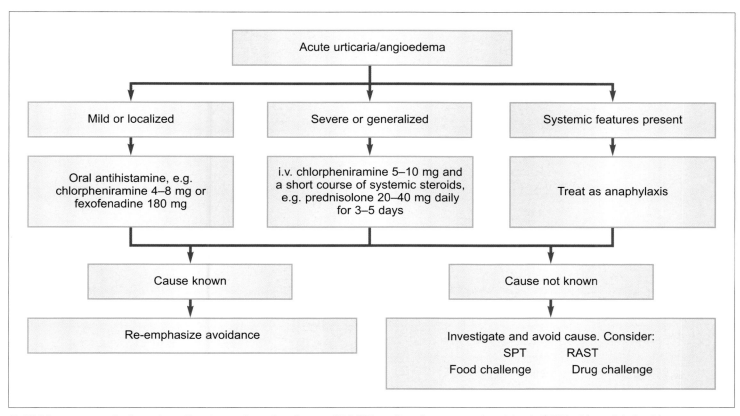

7.12 Management of acute urticaria and angioedema. (RAST, radio allergen sorbent test; SPT, skin prick test.)

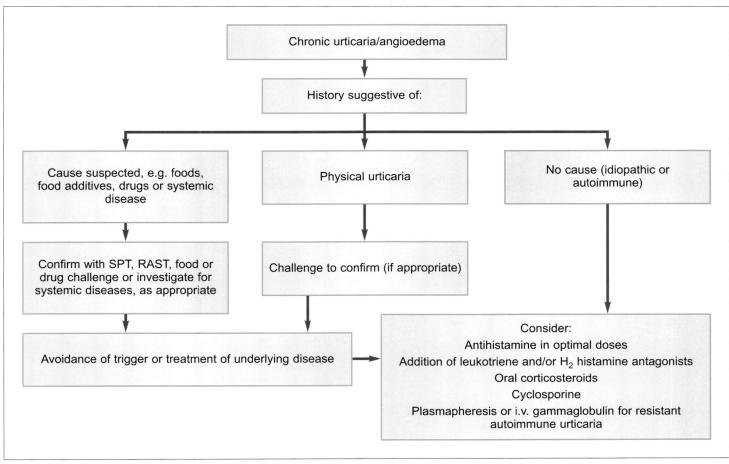

7.13 Management of chronic urticaria and angioedema. (RAST, radio allergen sorbent test; SPT, skin prick test.)

Chapter 8

Food allergy

Epidemiology

Adverse reactions to food, in which the pathogenesis involves an immunological response to food components, are termed 'food hypersensitivity reactions'. This is considered synonymous with food allergy. In contrast, food intolerance is an abnormal non-immunological reaction to an ingested food that may be pharmacological, toxic, or metabolic. It is estimated that food allergy occurs in 1–2% of adults, and 8% of children 6 years of age or under. Of that group of children, however, only about 3% have clinically-proven allergic reactions to foods (**8.1**).

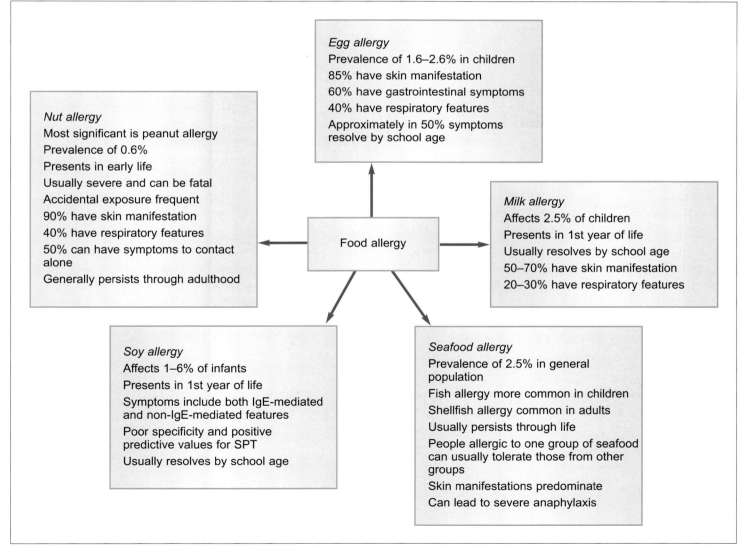

Egg allergy
Prevalence of 1.6–2.6% in children
85% have skin manifestation
60% have gastrointestinal symptoms
40% have respiratory features
Approximately in 50% symptoms resolve by school age

Nut allergy
Most significant is peanut allergy
Prevalence of 0.6%
Presents in early life
Usually severe and can be fatal
Accidental exposure frequent
90% have skin manifestation
40% have respiratory features
50% can have symptoms to contact alone
Generally persists through adulthood

Milk allergy
Affects 2.5% of children
Presents in 1st year of life
Usually resolves by school age
50–70% have skin manifestation
20–30% have respiratory features

Food allergy

Soy allergy
Affects 1–6% of infants
Presents in 1st year of life
Symptoms include both IgE-mediated and non-IgE-mediated features
Poor specificity and positive predictive values for SPT
Usually resolves by school age

Seafood allergy
Prevalence of 2.5% in general population
Fish allergy more common in children
Shellfish allergy common in adults
Usually persists through life
People allergic to one group of seafood can usually tolerate those from other groups
Skin manifestations predominate
Can lead to severe anaphylaxis

8.1 Most food allergies have their onset in infancy or early childhood. (SPT, skin prick test.)

Although most people have experienced a reaction to something they have eaten, only 1% of the adult population suffers from true immune reactions to food. A prospective study in Danish infants during the first 3 years of life found the prevalence to cow's milk allergy to be 2.2%. In another study from Great Britain, 7.4% of 18,582 respondents reported allergies to food additives. However, following double blind placebo controlled food challenges (DBPCFCs), investigators estimated a 0.01–0.23% prevalence of food additive intolerance. Although any food can elicit an allergic reaction, eight common foods account for over 90% of food allergies. These include milk, soy, tree nuts, peanuts, eggs, wheat, fish, and shellfish (**8.2–8.4**). While allergies to milk, soy, eggs, and wheat are likely to resolve, allergies to peanuts, tree nuts, fish, and shellfish are more likely to persist.

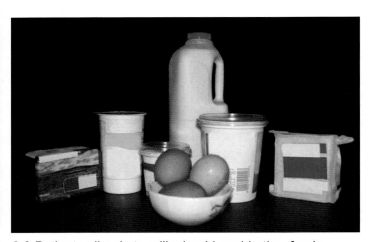

8.2 Patients allergic to milk should avoid other foods containing milk protein. These include butter, artificial butter, butter solids/fat, caramel colour, caramel flavouring, casein, cheese, cream, curds, flavouring, high protein flour, lactate, lactic acid, lactalbumin, lactalbumin phosphate, lactoferrin, lactaglobulin, lactose, margarine, buttermilk, milk fat, milk protein, milk solids, skim milk, powdered milk, dried milk, dry milk solids, sour milk solids, hydrolyzed milk protein, sour cream, whey, and yogurt. Egg white, especially raw or poorly cooked, causes more severe allergy than egg yolk. Patients allergic to egg should also avoid egg substitutes, egg shampoo, binders and fillers, bread, cakes, desserts, baked goods, and certain seasonings. Those allergic to oak pollen, ragweed, and the goosefoot family of weeds, may cross-react with eggs, when these pollens are in season.

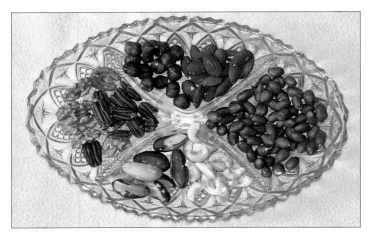

8.3 The most common allergenic nuts are cashew, almond, walnut, hazel, and brazil nuts. Some people have allergies to multiple nuts. Peanuts are a relatively common cause of allergies. However, they belong to legumes (vegetables), and are not nuts. If sensitive to nuts, it is important to avoid other nut-related products, such as chopped nuts, nut oils, nut spreads and paste, noisette, marzipan (if allergic to almonds), praline, and margarine (as it may contain nut oil).

8.4 Populations that consume or process large quantities of seafood tend to have the highest prevalence of seafood allergy. The fish commonly known to cause allergic reactions include cod, salmon, trout, herring, sardines, bass, swordfish, halibut, and tuna. Shellfish commonly known to cause allergic reactions include shrimp, crab, crayfish, lobster, oysters, clams, scallops, mussels, squid, and snails. The foods that contain fish/shellfish include Worcestershire sauce, Caesar salad, caviar, roe (fish eggs), and imitation seafood as is often used in sushi.

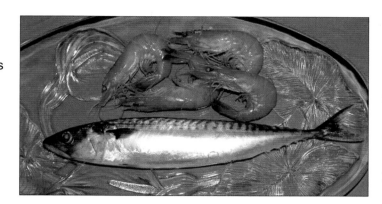

Pathophysiology of food allergy

Allergic reaction to foods is IgE or non-IgE mediated. Food allergens are typically glycoproteins which bind to the high-affinity IgE receptors. Subsequent allergen exposure leads to cross-linking of the food allergen-specific IgE on mast cells. This, then, leads to their degranulation and releasing histamine, PGs and LTs, resulting in clinical symptoms (**8.5**). Food allergens are generally water soluble and are resistant to proteolysis (*Table 8.1*). Closely related foods frequently contain allergens that have an immunological cross-reaction.

Allergic eosinophilic gastroenterocolitis appears to be due to repeated and severe IgE-mediated mucosal reactions to multiple foods. This leads to repeated early- and late-phase reactions in the GI mucosa. The pathogenesis of food protein enteropathy is not clear. These are more common in infants and resolve with age. IgM- and IgA-containing B-cells are increased in the *lamina propria* of patients with this condition, although this condition is not related to gliadin sensitivity.

Table 8.1 Food allergens

Food	Allergens
Cod fish	Gad C1
Shrimp	Tropomyosin (Pen a1, Pen il, Met e1)
Peanut	Ara h1
	Ara h2
	Ara h3
Soyabean	Trypsin inhibitor
	Thiol protease
	Conglycinin
Egg	Gal d1 (ovomucoid)
	Gal d2 (ovalbumin)
	Gal d3 (ovotransferrin)
	Gal d4 (lyzozyme)
Milk	α casein
	β lactoglobulin
	α lactalbumin
Brazil nut	Ber M 1
Rice	Ory S 1 (α amylase inhibitor)
Mustard	Sin a 1
	Bra j 1

Food allergens are usually proteins or glycoproteins with a molecular weight between 10 and 40 kDa. They are usually resistant to denaturation by heat and degradation by proteases. In infants, the majority of allergy is due to milk or soy. In adults, the most common food allergens are peanuts, crustacea, fish, and egg. In eggs, albumin has been found to be more allergenic than yolk

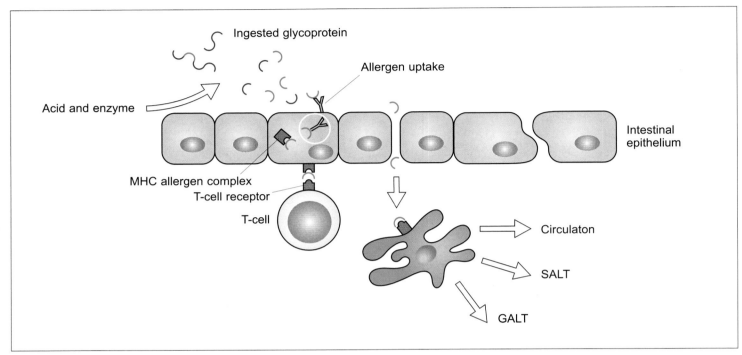

8.5 Immunologically active allergen glycoproteins are taken up by the intestinal mucosal cells. These allergen are processed and presented by the MHC complexes to the T-cells. In the normal situation, antigen presentation should suppress further immune response. However, in sensitized individuals there is an allergic response. Release of cytokines leads to loosening of the tight junctions between the intestinal epithelial cells, leading to a paracellular allergen inflow. Dendritic cells in the gut carry this allergen to the gut associated lymphoid organs. The non-GI manifestations tend to be IgE mediated. Here, helper T-cells activate B-cells, which in turn secrete allergen-specific IgE. The antibody circulates, becoming stationed on mast cells throughout the body, which are then ready to be triggered by allergen. (GALT, gut associated lymphod tissue; MHC, major histocompatibility complex; SALT, skin associated lymphoid tissue.)

Clinical features

Food allergy typically involves the skin, respiratory system, and GI tract (**8.6**).

Cutaneous reactions

Cutaneous reactions are the most common food allergic response. Symptoms range from urticaria and angioedema, to exacerbation of AD. Food allergy accounts for up to 20% of cases of acute urticaria and angioedema, and is mediated by IgE specific to food protein. Lesions usually occur within 1 hour after ingestion of, or contact with, the causal food (**8.7**). AD is a highly pruritic chronic inflammatory skin condition that commonly presents during early infancy and childhood. Food allergens induce skin rashes in 40% of

children with moderate to severe AD. Infants and children with food allergies generally have a positive skin test or allergen-specific IgE directed towards various foods, especially eggs, milk, soy, and peanut. Dermatitis herpetiformis (DH) is an immune-mediated blistering skin disease with an associated, often asymptomatic, gluten-sensitive enteropathy. The disorder is associated with a specific non-IgE-mediated immune sensitivity to gluten. Characteristic skin lesions found in patients with DH are extremely itchy grouped vesicles most frequently located on extensor surfaces. Most patients (as many as 80%) respond to gluten-free diet with control of their skin disease.

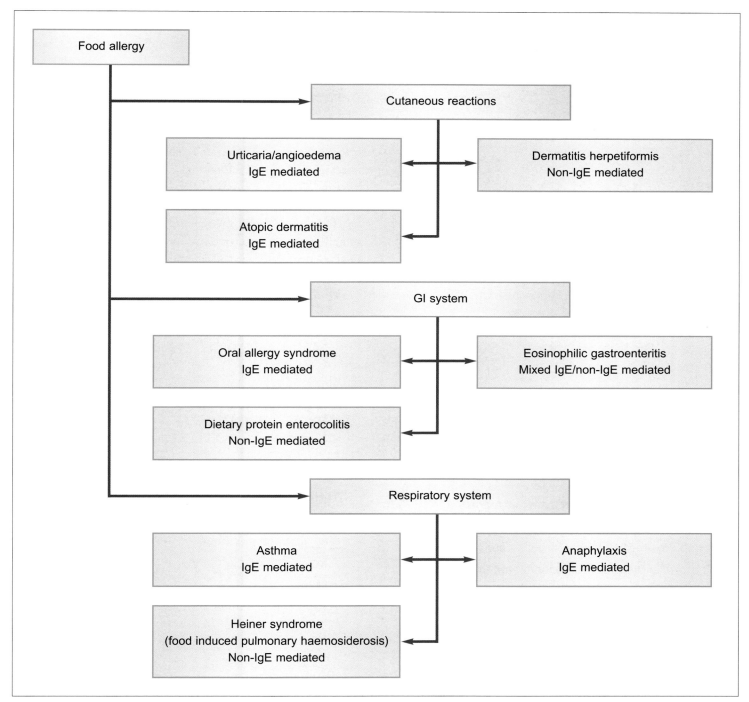

8.6 Food allergies could involve the GI system, the respiratory system, and the skin. They are either due to IgE-mediated mechanisms or due to non-IgE-mediated immune mechanisms.

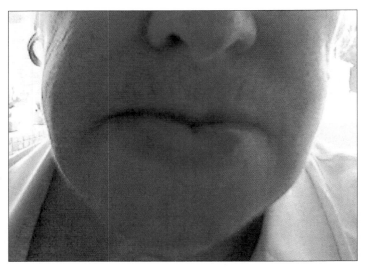

8.7 This patient with known IgE-mediated allergy to fish, had an acute allergic reaction with angioedema and swelling of the lips, mouth, and tongue, following inadvertent ingestion of fish. (The picture was taken by the patient as an aid to the diagnosis.)

Respiratory manifestations

Upper respiratory tract involvement causes laryngeal oedema, which may be life threatening. Wheezing is common in severe allergic reactions to food, but chronic asthma is rarely due to food allergy.

Gastrointestinal manifestations

The GI manifestation of food allergy could be either IgE mediated or non-IgE-mediated. Oral allergy syndrome is an IgE-mediated condition affecting the lips, mouth, and pharynx (*Table 8.2*). Individuals with this syndrome usually have a history of birch pollen sensitive seasonal allergic rhinitis. The other manifestations include eosinophilic gastroenteropathies, which include eosinophilic oeso-phagitis, gastroenterocolitis, and gastritis (*Table 8.3*). Dietary protein enterocolitis manifests in early infancy and the common triggers include cow's milk and soy protein (*Table 8.4*). This is not IgE mediated, as SPT and RAST are characteristically negative. This condition usually resolves by age 1–2 years.

Table 8.2 Oral allergy syndrome (pollen food syndrome)

- Oral pruritus
- Angioedema of lips, tongue, palate
- Rarely can lead to severe systemic reactions
- History of SAR
- Symptoms more frequent in pollen season
- The causal proteins are concentrated in the peel of some fruits
- Cooked form does not induce symptoms
- SPT characteristically positive

SAR, seasonal allergic rhinitis; SPT, skin prick test

Table 8.3 Clinical features of eosinophilic gastroenteropathies

- Nausea
- Dysphagia
- Abdominal pain
- Vomiting and diarrhoea
- Protein losing enteropathy
- Failure to thrive
- Ascitis due to serosal involvement

Table 8.4 Clinical features of dietary protein enteropathy

• Protracted diarrhoea	• Oedema
• Vomiting	• Ascites
• Malabsorbtion	• Anaemia
• Failure to thrive	

Diagnosis

The diagnostic approach for suspected food allergy begins with a detailed history and careful physical examination. The history should include the quantity of the suspect food ingested and the duration between ingestion and the development of symptoms. It should also include information about whether the ingested food has caused similar symptoms in the past, and whether there are any other co-existent factors required to induce the reaction. Diet cards are used as an adjunct to medical history. Patients are advised to keep chronological records of all the foods ingested over a specified period, and record any symptoms experienced by the patient.

The diagnosis of food allergy is based on standardized oral challenges (*Table 8.5*). Exceptions are high levels of specific IgE to eggs (>6 kUl/l), peanuts (>15 kUl/l), fish (>20 kUl/l), and milk (>32 kUl/l), reaching a 95% predictive positive value. RAST inhibition tests are useful to identify masked allergens in foods. Several studies observed that in infants and young children, low food-specific IgE levels were associated with positive food challenge outcomes. For egg allergy, a level of 2 kU_A/L or above in children younger than 2 years had 95% positive predictive value, whereas for milk, a level of 5 kU_A/L in infants younger than 1 year had 95% positive predictive value.

The diagnosis of non-IgE-mediated food allergy is difficult. Patch testing is typically used for diagnosis of delayed contact hypersensitivity reactions in which T-cells play a prominent role. In young children with challenge-proven milk allergy, SPTs were positive in 67% of the cases with acute-onset reactions (under 2 hours) to milk challenge, whereas patch tests tended to be negative. Patch tests were positive in 89% of children with delayed-onset reactions (25–44 hours). However, SPTs were frequently negative, indicating that the combination of patch testing and detection of IgE (with SPT or RAST) could enhance the accuracy of diagnosing food allergy, and may eliminate the need for oral food challenges.

Certain uncommon food hypersensitivity reactions (e.g. GI bleeding, milk-induced pulmonary disease [Heiner syndrome], and protein-losing enteropathy) are mediated totally, or partially, by IgG antibodies (*Table 8.6*). The mere presence of IgG antibodies in the circulation, however, is a normal physiologic phenomenon and indicates exposure. Only in certain cases, high titres may explain the immunological basis of a non-IgE-mediated reaction. Serum food-specific IgG antibody titres can be measured by radio-, enzyme-, or fluorescent-immunoassays that have better reproducibility than the previously used techniques of precipitation, haemagglutination, or complement fixation. Other investigations, such as lymphocyte proliferation assays, merely reflect exposure to food in the diet, and are not useful tools in differentiating between individuals with food allergy or without.

Table 8.5 Investigations for food allergy

- Blood eosinophils
- Serum total IgE
- Food specific IgE
- Basophil histamine assays
- Skin prick testing
- Intra-dermal skin tests
- Diet diary
- Elimination diet
- Food challenge:
- Open food challenge
- Single blinded food challenge
- Double blinded placebo controlled food challenge

Table 8.6 Investigations for differentiating the various GI manifestations of food allergy

Disorder	Key investigations	Other tests
Oral allergy syndrome	SPT	RAST
		Oral food challenge
Eosinophilic enteropathies	Elimination diet	SPT
	Biopsy	RAST
		Oral food challenge
Dietary protein enteropathy	Elimination diet	SPT
	Biopsy	RAST
		Oral food challenge

RAST, radio allergen sorbent test; SPT, skin prick test

Treatment

The therapy for food allergy is limited to dietary vigilance and the ability to treat the allergic reactions, if they occur. The only available therapy for food allergy is avoidance of the suspect food (**8.8**). Therapy in infants with cow's milk allergy usually involves selection of a hydrolyzed milk formula. Food cross-reactions occur within so-called botanical food families, and if a person is allergic to one food, then the development of allergies to other foods within the same food family is likely (*Table 8.7*). Hence, food avoidance advice should also include cross-reacting foods. The treatment of choice for food-induced anaphylaxis is intramuscular epinephrine. Promising new immunotherapy interventions are being investigated, but these are still in the early stages of development (*Table 8.8*).

Table 8.7 Cross-reacting allergens

Food allergen	Cross-reacting foods
Silver birch/hazel proteins	Parsnips, oranges, tomatoes, apples, pears, potatoes, onions, carrots, celery, hazel nut
Grass pollen	Peaches, plums, apricots, cherries
Mugwort pollen	Celery, peanuts, kiwi fruit, apples
Ragweed pollen	Bananas, watermelon, honeydew melon
Peanuts, soybeans	Legumes
Wheat	Other cereals
Latex	Bananas, chestnut, avocados, papaya, pineapple, kiwi fruit
Eggs	Chicken meat
Cow's milk	Beef, goat's milk
Beef	Lamb
Fish	Other fish

Pollen allergy can be associated with allergy to fruits, nuts, and vegetables and this is exemplified by the oral allergy syndrome. This is due to the presence of cross-reactive IgE antibodies. For example, the major birch pollen allergen, Bet v 1, has homology with allergens in apple, pear, celery, carrot, and potato

Table 8.8 Immunomodulatory therapies for food allergy, that might become available in the near future

- Anti-IgE
- Mutated allergen protein immunotherapy: the major safety concern regarding food allergen immunotherapy has been addressed by engineering 'hypoallergenic' forms of major allergenic food proteins. These mutated ('engineered') major food proteins have lost their ability to bind to IgE but retain the ability to interact with T-cells. Initial studies have shown desensitization; the modified Ara h2 protein suppressed synthesis of Ara h2-IgE and resulted in significantly decreased symptoms on oral peanut challenge compared with a control group treated with native Ara h2
- Peptide immunotherapy
- Immunostimulatory sequences
- Probiotic

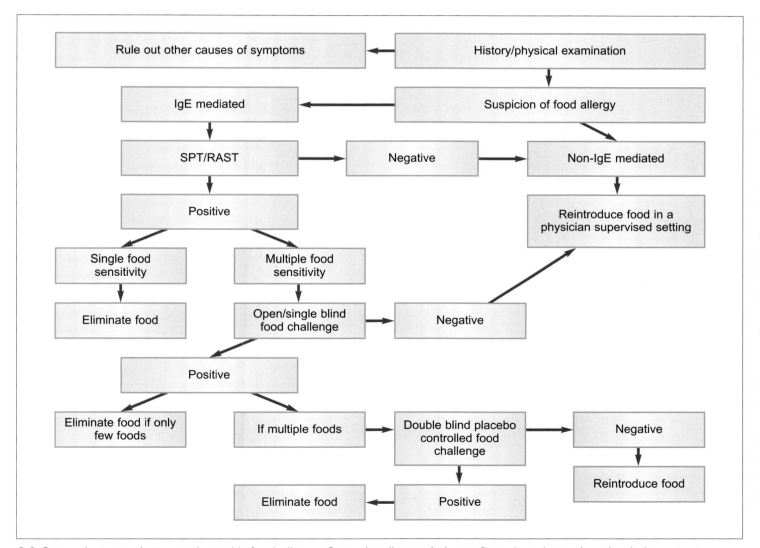

8.8 General approach to a patient with food allergy. Once the diagnosis is confirmed, patient education is important and advice regarding avoidance and steps to be taken in an emergency should be clearly defined. Patient should be evaluated for compliance. (RAST, radio allergen sorbent test; SPT, skin prick test.)

Chapter 9

Insect allergy

Introduction

The stinging insects are from the order Hymenoptera, which includes the families Vespidae (wasps, hornets, and yellow jackets), Apidae (bees), and Formicidae (ants) (**9.1–9.4**). In the USA, insect bite allergy is responsible for at least 50 fatalities per year, and as many as two million people are allergic to the venom of stinging insects. The incidence of systemic sting reactions in the general population range from 0.3–7.5%, depending on the population. Systemic sting reactions have been reported in 22–43%, and large local reactions in 31–38% of beekeepers. In children, these reactions are usually limited to cutaneous signs, with urticaria and angioedema; adults more commonly have airway obstruction or hypotension. Compared with adults, children have a higher frequency of isolated cutaneous actions to insect stings and a lower frequency of vascular symptoms and anaphylactic shock. With regards to fire ants, as many as 50% of individuals report large local reactions, and up to 1% of fire ant stings may result in anaphylaxis. There is significant cross-reactivity between allergens of these insects (*Table 9.1*).

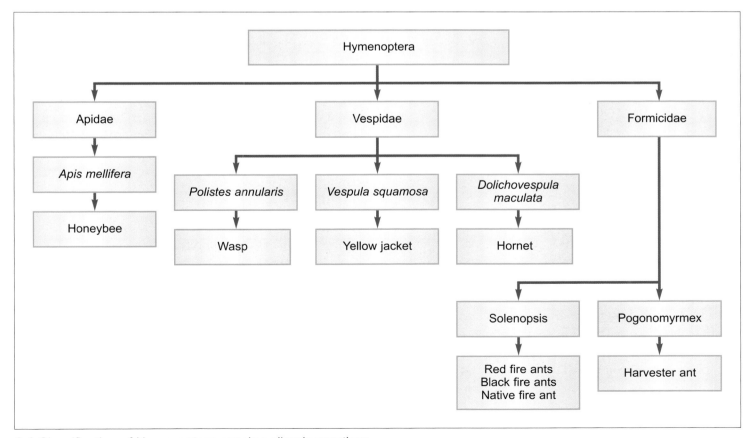

9.1 Classification of Hymenoptera causing allergic reactions.

9.2 A honeybee (*Apis mellifera*) has a barbed stinger, which usually remains in the skin following a sting. A honeybee dies after stinging because it eviscerates itself while leaving its stinger and venom sac behind. Bumblebees, which

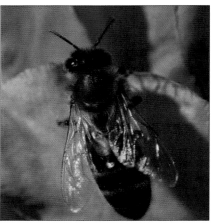

are generally larger, hairier, and more colourful than honeybees, have a stinger with fewer barbs and a stronger attachment. Consequently, bumblebees can sting repeatedly and do not die after stinging. Although bee and wasp venom varies from species to species, all venom is composed primarily of proteins, peptides, and amines. Toxic components include phospholipase, histamine, bradykinin, acetylcholine, dopamine, and serotonin. In addition, mast cell degranulating peptide and mastoparan are peptides that can cause degranulation of mast cells, and result in an anaphylactoid reaction. Depending on the location and number of bee stings received, severe anaphylaxis can be precipitated that can be life threatening. (Courtesy of Hania Arentsen.)

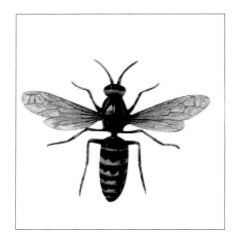

9.3 Reactions to hornet (*Vespa cabro*) stings are similar to bee stings. In a sensitized individual, this can lead to severe anaphylaxis.

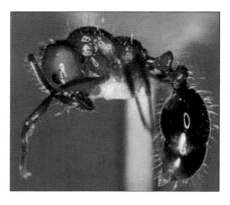

9.4 Fire ants (*Solenopsis invicta*) inflict a sting, which causes a small blister or pustule to form at the site of each sting after several hours. 95% of fire ant venom is water-insoluble and non-proteinaceous and contains dialkylpiperidine haemolytic factors. These haemolytic factors induce the release of histamine and other vasoactive amines from mast cells, resulting in a sterile pustule at the sting site. These alkaloids are not immunogenic, but their toxicity to the skin is believed to cause the pustules to form. Systemic reactions can be fatal. (Peter Green, Department of Primary Industries and Fisheries, Queensland, Australia.)

Clinical features

The normal reaction of the skin to a bee or wasp sting consists of a painful, sometimes itchy, local weal, developing up to a 2 cm diameter, surrounded by a swelling involving subcutaneous tissue several centimetres in diameter. The local dermal reaction results from a non-immunological reaction to the potent pharmacological and enzyme constituents of the venom. The local reaction to a fire ant sting is unique in that the uncomplicated local reaction evolves into a sterile pustule. This sterile pustule appears to result from the effects of the piperidine alkaloids which constitute 95% of the venom.

Allergy is a harmful physiological event that is mediated through immunological reactions. Large local reactions involve oedema at the sting site, with a diameter exceeding 10 cm and lasting over 24 hours (**9.5**). Systemic reactions vary greatly in severity, and they can be classified in four grades (**9.6**). Patients with mastocytosis are particularly prone to anaphylactoid reactions following insect sting. Patients on beta blockers and angiotensin-converting enzyme inhibitors appear to be at a higher risk of anaphylaxis. Other reactions have been described, including serum sickness-like illness, fever with neurological symptoms, and reversible renal disease.

Table 9.1 Insect sting allergens

	Allergens	Common name	Molecular weight (kD)
Honey bee	Api M I	Phospholipase A2	16
	Api M II	Hyaluronidase	39
	Api M III	Melittin	3
	Api M IV	Acid phosphatase	43
		Apamin	
		Peptide 401	
Wasps, hornets, yellow jackets	Dol M I	Phospholipase A1	34
	Dol M II	Hyaluronidase	39
	Dol M III	Acid phosphatase	43
	Dol M V	Antigen 5	23
		Kinin	
		Mastoparan	
Fire ants	Sol i I	Phospholipase A1	37
	Sol i II	-	32
	Sol i III	Antigen 5 family	23
	Sol i IV	-	20

There is extensive cross-reactivity of allergens between yellow jackets and hornets and moderate cross-reactivity between these insects and wasps. (Adapted from WHO nomenclature [1988]. *J Allergy Clin Immunol*, **82**:818)

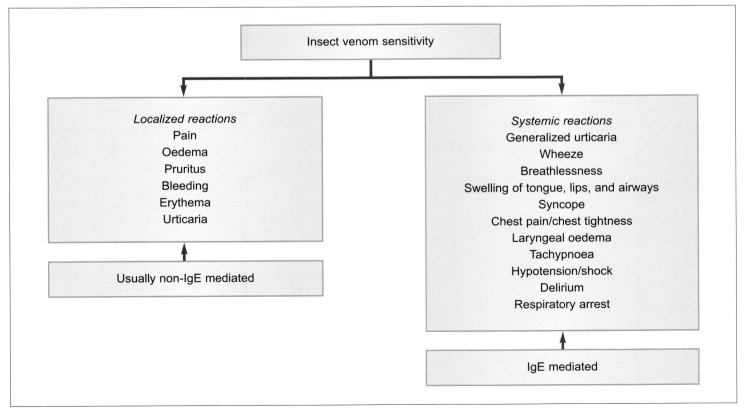

9.5 Clinical features of reactions to insect stings.

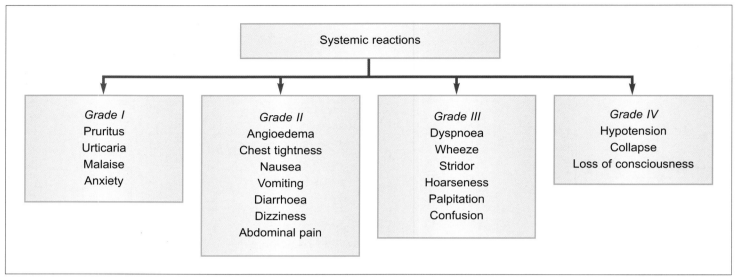

9.6 Systemic reactions can be classified into different grades based on the severity of the reaction.

Diagnosis

A clinical history characteristic of an allergic reaction is very important in the diagnosis of insect venom sensitivity. This can be demonstrated by the presence of venom-specific IgE by RAST and by SPTs (*Table 9.2*). SPTs are more sensitive and specific than the *in vitro* RAST. Commercially available insect venom test kits include honeybee, wasps, yellow jackets, yellow hornet, and white-faced hornet. Honeybee venoms can be used for the diagnosis of bumblebee sensitivity. Fire ant venom is not commercially available and, hence, whole-body extracts of fire ants are used instead. Some centres perform sting challenges with the live insect. However studies have shown that 25% of patients challenged with yellow jacket stings, and 52% of patients challenged with honeybee stings developed anaphylactic reactions. Therefore sting challenges are not considered a necessary criterion for instituting immunotherapy.

Table 9.2 Diagnostic features of insect allergy

- History suggestive of allergic reaction
- Positive SPTs for venom-specific IgE
- RAST for venom-specific IgE
- Sting challenges
- Live insects

RAST, radio allergen sorbent test; SPT, skin prick test

Treatment

Most patients with insect bites or stings only need symptomatic treatment for the symptoms of pain and itching. Unlike other insects that sting, the honeybee leaves its stinger behind. Proper removal of this stinger following a honeybee sting can help prevent worsening symptoms. The local reactions, such as pain, redness, and itching, can be treated with cold compresses, analgesics, and oral antihistamines (**9.7**). Antibiotics may be required if the wound is infected.

Some patients develop large localized reactions, which may require systemic corticosteroids, in addition to antihistamines and analgesics. Severe reactions should be managed in a hospital similar to anaphylactic reactions. Intramuscular or subcutaneous epinephrine should be administered in emergency.

Further treatment includes intravenous fluids, systemic corticosteroids, and antihistamines, as well as nebulized β2-agonists for chest tightness and wheeze. Immunotherapy should be instituted for patients with allergic reactions to Hymenoptera (*Table 9.3*, p102). Treatment extracts for allergen immunotherapy are commercially available (**9.8**). Patients allergic to Hymenoptera should be advised to avoid these insects, and instructed how to take the necessary steps if they are stung. Patients with severe reaction should be provided with an Epipen to keep handy in an emergency, and educated about the use of Epipen. These patients should also be provided with a medic alert bracelet.

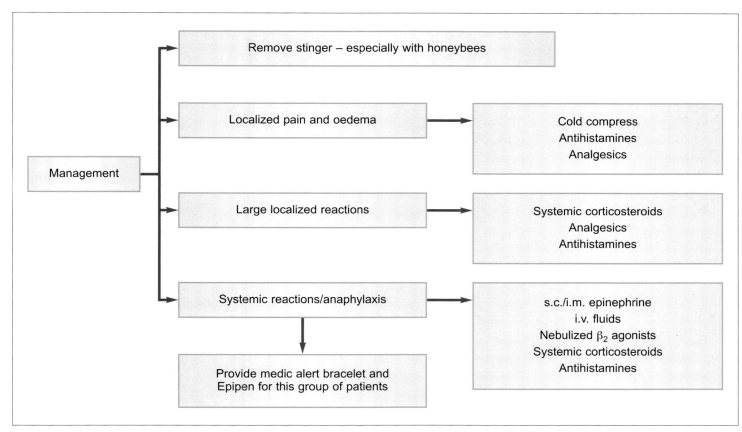

9.7 Following a Hymenoptera sting, it is crucial to remove any stinger that may remain because the venom sac can continue to exude venom into the skin. While honeybees are most well known for leaving stingers behind, other members of the Hymenoptera order may also leave a stinger behind in some instances. Removal of the stinger should be accomplished by sweeping the dull blade of a butter knife or edge of a credit card across the skin at an angle almost parallel to the surface. This prevents additional venom squeezing out of the sac. Removal with tweezers should be avoided, as this may compress the venom sac and result in the injection of additional venom into the skin. Patients developing severe reactions should be managed in the hospital and treatment instituted for anaphylaxis. This group of patients should be provided with a medic alert bracelet and Epipen for use in an emergency in case they have another sting. Immunotherapy is performed for adults with systemic allergic reactions and children with reactions more severe than generalized urticaria or cutaneous angioedema. Venom immunotherapy is rarely indicated for treatment of large local reactions or isolated urticaria.

Specific injection immunotherapy (SIT) has a role in the management of Hymenoptera sensitivity and allergic rhinitis. SIT also seems to be effective in asthmatic patients with cat allergy. The major drawback is that most asthmatics are sensitized to multiple allergens, and SIT addresses only the allergen used in the injection. There is also an increased risk of severe adverse reactions. However, the answer might lie in using epitopes, instead of whole allergens. Epitopes eliminate any of the dangers generated by the whole antigen, such as IgE-mediated anaphylaxis. Immunization with epitopes is actually more efficient than injections of whole allergen in the induction of peripheral T-cell tolerance. The future of immunotherapy may lie in the identification of immunostimulatory DNA sequence that can activate a specific pathway towards a Th1 response. This could be the basis for the use of a vaccine in the management of allergy. (i.m. intramuscular; i.v., intravenous; s.c., subcutaneous.)

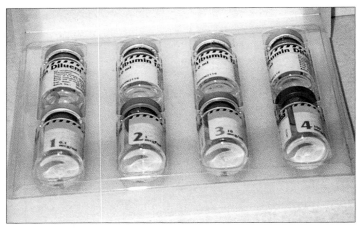

9.8 Treatment extract for allergen-specific immunotherapy for wasp venom is commercially available in four gradually increasing concentrations. Treatment is started with the lowest concentration vial, and with a small dose. The dose and concentrations are gradually increased until maintenance dose is reached.

Table 9.3 Allergen immunotherapy for insect allergy

- Immunotherapy aims to induce tolerance to the specific venom
- The exact mode of action of immunotherapy is not known
- The venom is injected subcutaneously in gradually increasing quantities at weekly intervals, until the maintenance dose is reached
- Thereafter, the injections are given at longer (4 weekly) intervals for 2–5 years
- The benefit continues after injections are discontinued
- In venom allergy, the evidence of effectiveness is excellent
- Immunotherapy can have serious adverse effects including anaphylaxis
- Minor reactions usually respond well to antihistamine
- Immunotherapy should only be performed where facilities for resuscitation are available

Avoidance

Avoidance is a key element in guarding against severe allergic reactions to insect stings. Simple steps to avoid attracting or provoking stinging insects when outdoors include: avoiding brightly coloured clothing or sweet-smelling cosmetics and shampoos; keeping food and garbage covered; wearing shoes to guard against stepping on insects; keeping arms and legs covered during activities that may expose the subject to stinging insects (such as gardening or hiking); refraining from swatting or crushing insects; and steering clear of areas where insects have nested.

Other insects

Unlike the group Hymenoptera, allergic reactions to other biting insects are infrequent. The most commonly reported reactions are to kissing bug (**9.9**). Allergic reactions to other insects and arthropods, such as spiders, chiggers, caterpillars, and scorpions, occasionally occur (**9.10–9.14**). Though the symptoms are predominantly due to their venom, allergic reactions do occur.

9.9 Kissing bug (or assasin bug, *Triatoma*) bite is painless and generally occurs on the uncovered parts of the body. Victims usually wake up with itching, swelling, and tachycardia. Depending on the patient's sensitivity, reactions to kissing bugs vary from mild to life threatening. A typical reaction is generally an intensely itchy, red, raised area that is more severe than a typical insect bite. It lasts about 1–2 days, but may last as long as 1 week. Other reactions can include groups of small blister-like bites with moderate swelling and little redness, very large reddened areas like hives that can be 5–15 cm across, chills, fever, and nausea. Severe reactions include swelling of the tongue and throat, lymphadenopathy, small blood-filled blisters, anaphylactic reactions causing wheeze and chest tightness, hypotension, and shock which can be lethal. (Courtesy of R Grantham, Oklahoma State University, USA.)

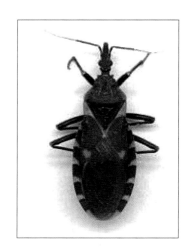

9.10 The black widow spider (*Latrodectus mactans*) (common in the USA) is common around wood piles, and is frequently encountered when homeowners carry firewood into the house. The female black widow is shiny black, usually with a reddish hourglass shape on the underside of her spherical abdomen. The bite of the female black widow spider may not always be felt at first, and besides slight local swelling, there is usually little evidence of a lesion. Two tiny red spots can sometimes be observed in the centre of the swollen area. Most of the time, pain at the site of the bite occurs immediately and becomes most intense after about 3 hours. An overall aching of the body, especially the legs, are common reactions. Headache, elevated blood pressure, nausea, and profuse perspiration may

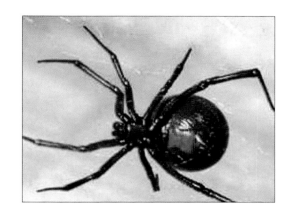

occur in severe cases. The condition is self-limiting and, in most cases, symptoms disappear in 2 or 3 days. Although most patients recover even without treatment, in up to 5% of patients, paralysis, convulsions, shock, and death occur. Young children, the elderly, persons with underlying hypertension, and pregnant women are considered to be at highest risk. (Courtesy of J Jackman, Texas Cooperative Extension, USA.)

9.11 The physical reaction to a brown recluse spider (*Loxosceles recluse*) bite depends on the amount of venom injected, and an individual's sensitivity to it. The symptoms may vary from no harm at all to a reaction that is very severe. Often there is a systemic reaction within 24–36 hours, characterized by restlessness, fever, chills, nausea, weakness, and joint pain. Where the bite occurs there is often tissue death and skin is sloughed off. Systemic illness, including mild haemolysis and mild coagulopathy, has been reported.

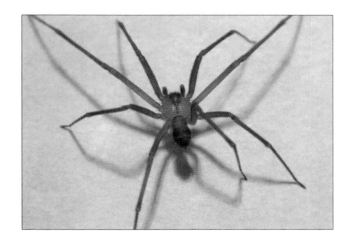

9.12 The full-grown larva of the Io caterpillar (*Automeris io*) is 5.7–6.5 cm long, and fairly easy to recognize. The head and body are yellowish green; thoracic legs and prolegs are red. There is a broad white line along each side, bordered above by a similar reddish line and below by a thinner (sometimes broken) reddish-purple line. Raised tubercles, each bearing a whorl of green branched spines, occur on each segment along the back. In contrast to bees and hornets, Io caterpillars bear specialized nettling or urticaceous setae or spines. These structures are hollow and contain toxins from poison-gland cells to which they are linked. The sting inflicted on humans is not from a deliberate attack by the caterpillar, but the result of contact, usually inadvertent, with toxin-bearing setae or spines. When brushed against, these structures break away, releasing toxins. In some cases, broken setae may penetrate the skin; in others, toxins spill out to spread on the surface of the skin.

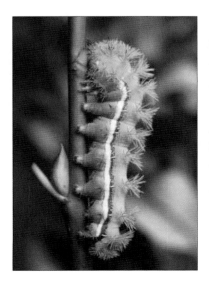

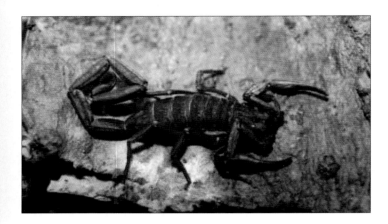

9.13 Scorpions (*Centrutoides gracils* illustrated) are nocturnal animals and, therefore, usually only emerge at night. Typical allergic reactions are: blurring of consciousness, unconsciousness, convulsions, fall in blood pressure, and shock; consequently, the threat of death may occur.

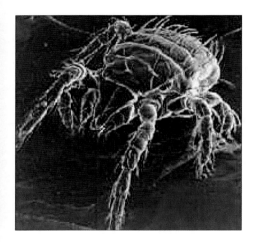

9.14 Chigger mites (*Trombicula* sp.) are unique among the many mite families in that only the larval stage feeds on vertebrate animals. Chigger bites itch so intensely and for so long a time because the chigger injects saliva into its victim after attaching to the skin. This saliva contains a powerful digestive enzyme that literally dissolves the skin cells it contacts. It is this liquefied tissue, never blood, that the chigger ingests and uses for food. The reactions induced by these mites are usually localized.

Chapter 10

Drug allergy

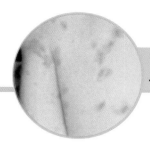

Introduction

Adverse drug reactions (ADRs) are any noxious, unintended, or undesired effects of a drug that occur at doses used in humans for prophylaxis, diagnosis, or treatment. ADRs account for 2–6% of all hospital admissions. The reaction rate to antibiotics is in the range of 1–8% for several classes of antibiotics, and non-steroidal anti-inflammatory drugs (NSAIDs) are common causes of rashes, especially urticaria. The most important drug-related risk factors for drug hyper-sensitivity concern the chemical properties and molecular weight of the drug (*Table 10.1*). Larger drugs with greater structural complexity (e.g. non-human proteins) are more likely to be immunogenic. Heterologous antisera, streptokinase, and insulin are examples of complex antigens capable of eliciting hyper-sensitivity reactions. The existence of specific factors that increase the risk of general adverse drug reactions include female gender, infection with HIV, herpes, asthma, systemic lupus erythematosus, and use of beta blockers.

Classification

Drug reactions can be classified as either predictable or unpredictable (**10.1**). Predictable reactions (Type A), or augmented reactions, are due to unknown pharmacological actions of the drug, and are usually dose related, occurring in otherwise normal individuals. These include over-dosage, side-effects, and interactions with other drugs. Unpredictable reactions (type B), or bizarre reactions, are dose independent, not related to the pharmacological actions of the drug, and may have a genetic basis. These may be further classified as immunological and non-immunological. Immunological drug eruptions are essentially based on the Gell and Coombs classification, but only a limited number of drug reactions fit into this classification (*Table 10.2*). Non-immunological mechanisms include: phototoxicity; pharmacological destabilization of mast cells; activation of complement in the absence of antibody; and toxicity of drug metabolites. Idiosyncratic reactions are a type of non-immunological unpredictable reactions, and are less common than pharmacological adverse reactions. Nevertheless, they are important because they can be serious and account for many deaths.

Table 10.1 Factors influencing drug reactions

- Chemical nature of the drug
- Size of the molecule
- Age/sex
- Genetic factors
- Use of multiple drugs
- Underlying disease like HIV/herpes/IMN
- Deranges renal and liver functions

HIV, human immunodeficiency virus; IMN, infectious mononucleosis

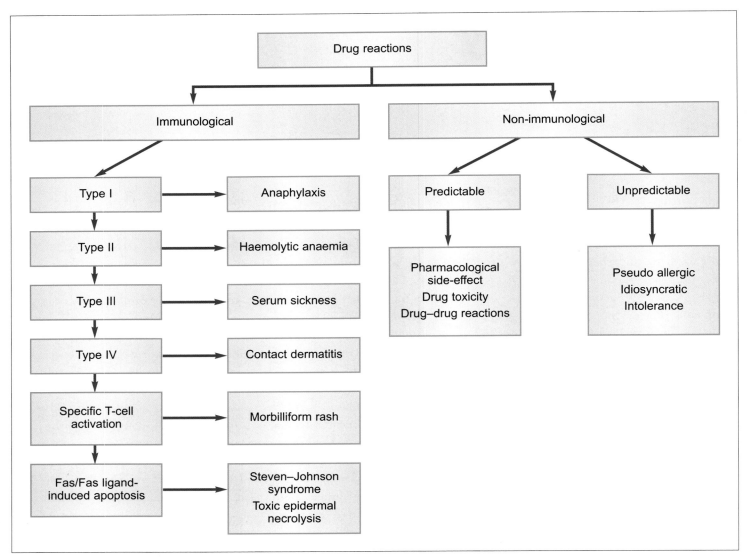

10.1 Classification of drug reactions.

Clinical features

A thorough physical examination is essential in the evaluation of cutaneous drug eruptions (**10.2**). Cutaneous drug reactions may be associated with systemic anaphylaxis, or with extensive muco-cutaneous exfoliation and multi-system involvement. Signs warranting discontinuation of the drugs are: mucous membrane erosions, blisters, confluent erythema, angioedema and tongue swelling, palpable purpura, skin necrosis, lymphadenopathy, and fever.

The skin lesions should be described based on their distribution and morphology (*Table 10.3*). The morphology of the lesions could provide a clue regarding the most likely culprit. Morbilliform or maculopapular exanthems are the most common patterns, appearing in 30–50% of cutaneous drug reactions. Morbilliform eruptions occur within 1 week

of beginning treatment, and last for 1–2 weeks. These do not always recur with re-challenge. The likely drugs should be discontinued, as continued administration may lead to confluence of lesions and generalized erythroderma, or exfoliative dermatitis. A morbilliform eruption is often the initial presentation of a more severe reaction, such as toxic epidermal necrolysis (TEN), hypersensitivity syndrome, and serum sickness. Urticaria is the mildest form of cutaneous skin reactions and, although quite a few drugs are implicated, it is important to note that certain drugs, such as salicylates, opiates, and radio contrast agents, can cause urticaria by non-immune mechanisms (**10.3**). Re-administration of the offending drug may lead to anaphylaxis due to IgE-mediated mechanisms. Drugs also

Table 10.2 Gell and Coombs classification of drug-induced hypersensitivity

Hypersensitivity reactions	Synonym	Immunological mechanism	Mediators of tissue injury and inflammation	Examples
Type 1	Immediate hypersensitivity	Mediated by drug-specific IgE antibodies	Vasoactive products of mast cells/basophils	Anaphylaxis, urticaria, angioedema
Type 2	Antibody-mediated cytotoxic hypersensitivity	Mediated by drug-specific IgM and IgG antibodies	Complement	Vasculitis
Type 3	Immune complex-mediated hypersensitivity	Mediated by drug-specific IgG and IgM antibodies	Complement	Serum sickness vasculitis
Type 4	Cell-mediated hypersensitivity	Drug-specific T-lymphocyte mediated reaction	Lymphokines and monokine	Contact sensitivity, maculopapular rash, morbilliform eruption, fixed drug eruption, photodrug reaction, exfoliative dermatitis, erythema multiforme, Stevens–Johnson syndrome, toxic epidermal necrolysis

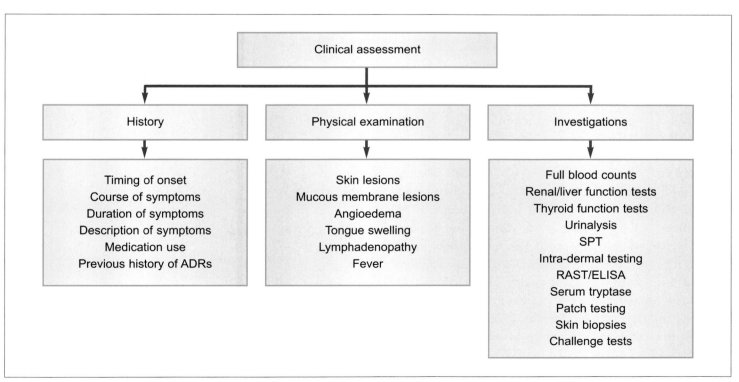

10.2 Assessment of adverse reactions to drugs (ADRs). (ELISA, enzyme-linked immunosorbent assay; RAST, radio allergen sorbent test; SPT, skin prick test.)

Table 10.3 Cutaneous manifestation of drug reactions

Cutaneous manifestation	Drugs implicated
Urticaria	Aspirin, NSAIDs, angiotensin-converting enzyme inhibitors, penicillin, cephalosporins, opiates, peptide hormones, radiocontrast dyes, vaccines
Maculopapular eruptions	Aspirin, NSAIDs, ampicillin, anticonvulsants, barbiturates, isoniazid, phenothiazines, quinalones, sulphonamides, thiazides, co-trimoxazole
Pemphigus	Penicillamine, gold, levodopa, heroin, penicillin, rifampin, phenylbutazone
Photosensitivity	Amiodarone, chlorpromazine, frusemide, quinalones, sulphonamides, tetracycline, thiazides
Fixed drug eruptions	Acetaminophen, penicillin, anticonvulsants, barbiturates, metronidazole, OCPs
Steven–Johnson syndrome, TEN	Sulphonamides, co-trimoxazole, tetracyclines, barbiturates, thiazetazone, phenytoin, carbamazepine, phenylbutazone
Vascullitis	Allopurinol, cimetidine, gold, phenytoin, quinalones, propyl-thio-uracil, thiazides, NSAIDs
Vesiculo-bullous eruptions	Aspirin, NSAIDs, barbiturates, frusemide, griseofulvin, penicillamine, penicillin, sulphonamides, thiazide

NSAIDs, non-steroidal anti-inflammatory drugs; OCPs, oral contraceptive pills; TEN, toxic epidermal necrolysis

cause chronic urticaria and aspirin frequently exacerbates this problem. Erythema multiforme is an acute self-limiting inflammatory disorder of the skin and mucous membrane associated with sore throat and malaise. Typically, there are target, iris, or bull's eye lesions, with a time course of <4 weeks.

Extensive lesions with mucous membrane involvement are called Steven–Johnson syndrome (SJS). The mortality rates have been reported to be as high as 5–15% for SJS. The more severe form of SJS is termed TEN. The discrimination between SJS and TEN is based on the extent of skin involvement. In SJS, there is detachment of <10% of epidermis, while TEN is associated with >30% involvement of the skin. The condition is characterized by confluent erythema followed by extensive areas of epidermal detachment, and there may be raised flaccid blisters, which spread with pressure. In cases of detachment of epidermis between 10–30%, it is considered as overlap between SJS and TEN. The epithelium of the airways and GI tract can also be involved. The presence of purpura and petichiae are often cutaneous stigmata of vasculitis.

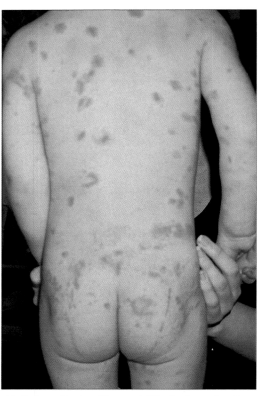

10.3 A patient with penicillin-induced urticaria.

Diagnosis

The most important aspect in the diagnosis of a drug reaction is the medical history. Although diagnostic tests exist, they are still of limited practical value for the clinician in evaluating a patient with suspected drug eruptions. SPTs are useful in IgE-mediated reactions. A positive SPT indicates that IgE antibodies to the drug are present, but a negative skin test does not exclude the absence of drug-specific IgE antibodies. Immediate skin testing is available for penicillins, cephalosporins, muscle relaxants, thiopentone, streptokinase, chymotrypsin, cisplatin, and insulin (**10.4**). Immunoassays such as RAST and ELISA can be used to detect IgE antibodies to aminoglycosides, sulphonamides, trimethoprim, insulin, and many β-lactam antibiotics. Serum tryptase estimation is employed to evaluate patients with suspected drug reaction. Tryptase is a protease found in mast cells and is released on mast cell degranulation. A raised tryptase does not establish the presence of drug-specific IgE antibodies, but is an indicator of mast cell mediator release. Skin biopsies are occasionally used to define specific histopathological lesions. It is useful in differentiating vasculitis and excluding bullous disease, not related to drug therapy, from SJS/TEN.

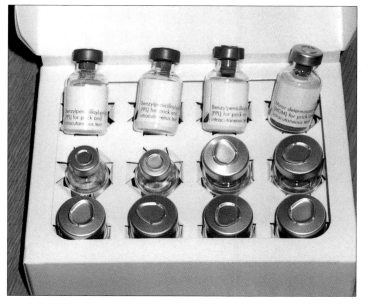

10.4 Diagnostic extracts (major and minor determinants) are commercially available for testing allergy to penicillin.

Management

The management of cutaneous drug eruptions involves identification and withdrawal of the drug, introduction of necessary supportive and suppressive treatment if the condition is severe, and considering alternative substitutes for the offending agent (**10.5**). Withdrawal of the drug is almost always prudent, and may immediately attenuate the reaction. In the case of mild type I reactions, such as urticaria and pruritus, antihistamines can be beneficial to suppress the symptoms with continuation of the treatment.

Certain cutaneous drug reactions, such as SJS, TEN, and some hypersensitivity reactions, need to be treated without delay because these medical emergencies are associated with considerable morbidity and mortality. The management and treatment of SJS and TEN are similar to treatment of burns with aggressive fluid management, nutritional support, and antibiotics. The role of corticosteroids is controversial in the management of SJS and TEN.

There are three approaches available to provide pharmacotherapy for the underlying condition in patients with cutaneous drug reactions. The first is the most safe and efficient method wherein an unrelated alternative drug is chosen. This situation works well with antibiotics. The second option is to choose a medication not identical but potentially cross-reacting with the offending drug, for example cephalosporins for penicillin-sensitive patients. However, this should be done with caution, as immunological cross-reactivity between penicillins and cephalosporin may be as high as 15–25% for first generation cephalosporins, but appears to be lower for third generation cephalosporins. Potentially cross-reacting drugs should not be reintroduced, even in graded doses, for patients who have experienced SJS/TEN. The third choice is drug desensitization. It is possible sometimes to readminister the offending drug in a patient who has had a drug eruption. Re-administration is usually done with gradually escalating doses of the offending agent. Certain factors need to be taken into account when re-administering the medication. For IgE-mediated reactions, re-administration can precipitate anaphylaxis, while in exfoliative conditions, SJS and TEN, this is contraindicated.

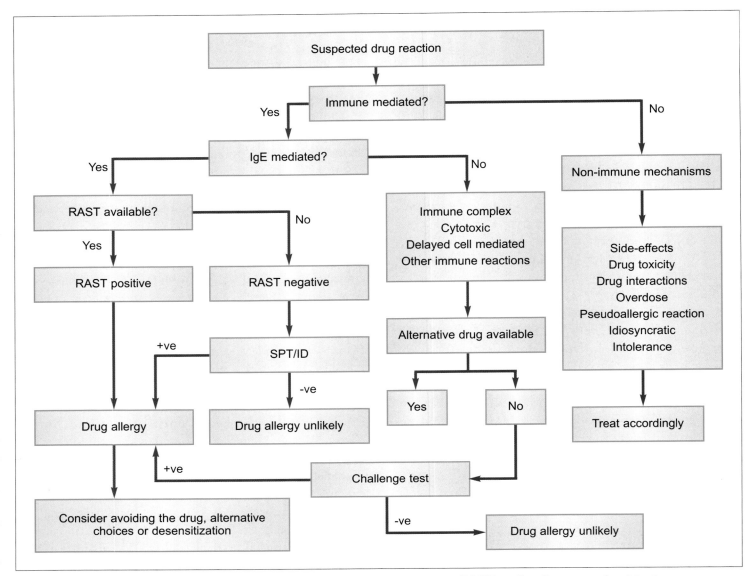

10.5 Diagnostic approach to suspected drug allergy. (ID, intra-dermal test; RAST; radio allergen sorbent test; SPT, skin prick test.)

Latex allergy

Latex is a natural product which comes from the light milky fluid that is extracted from the rubber tree. This milky fluid is often modified during the manufacturing process to form a latex mixture. A person can be allergic to the latex, or the mixture, or both. Incidence of latex allergy is now about 25% in health care workers, and 2–6% in the general population, due to the increased use of latex to protect ourselves from infections and other diseases (*Table 10.4*). The highest prevalence of latex allergy (20–68%) is found in patients with spina bifida or congenital urogenital abnormalities. Sensitization in these patients apparently follows multiple urinary tract, rectal, and thecal procedures, as well as multiple surgeries during early childhood. Patients with spina bifida also may have a genetic predisposition for latex sensitization.

There are three different types of reactions to natural rubber latex (**10.6**). They are irritation, delayed hypersensitivity (allergic CD) and immediate hypersensitivity (anaphylactic symptoms). The diagnosis of latex allergy includes serum IgE levels, specific IgE, SPT, and patch testing for CD. Treatment in an acute scenario is similar to the management of acute anaphylactic reactions. Latex-free

Table 10.4 Risk factors for latex sensitivity

- Patients with spina bifida
- Patients with congenital genito-urinary abnormalities
- Health care workers
- Rubber industry workers
- Atopic individuals
- Patients who have had multiple surgucal procedures
- Patients with certain food allergies

resuscitation equipment must be available and routine care should employ non-latex supplies. Prevention and taking adequate precautions are important in avoiding further reactions (**10.7**). Patients allergic to latex are at times sensitive to certain foods, including bananas, avocados, chestnuts, apples, carrots, celery, papaya, kiwi, potatoes, tomatoes, and melons. Food sensitivity of those allergic to latex may possibly also include pears, peaches, cherries, pineapple, strawberries, figs, grapes, apricots, passion fruit, rye, hazel nuts, walnuts, soy beans, and peanuts. Type IV hyper-sensitivity is best treated with patient education to avoid further exposure.

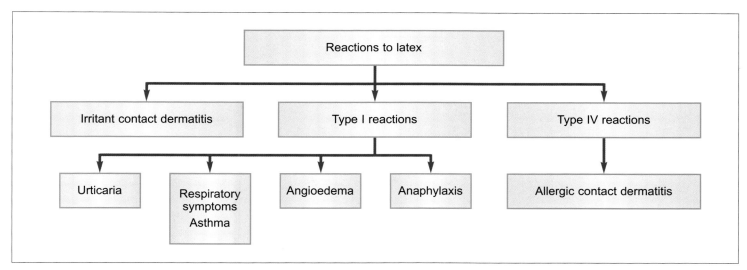

10.6 Irritant dermatitis is due to mechanical disruption of the skin due to rubbing of the gloves and accounts for the majority of latex-induced reactions. This is not immune mediated. The second most common is contact dermatitis. The least common, but potentially serious reactions, are the IgE-mediated type I reactions.

10.7 Avoidance of contact with natural rubber latex.

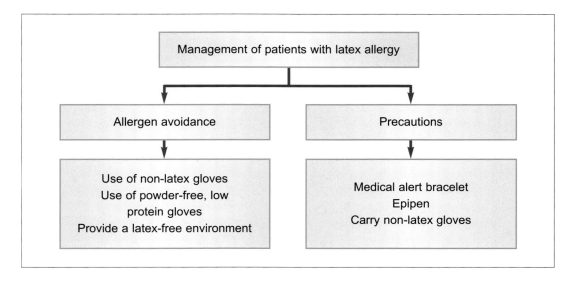

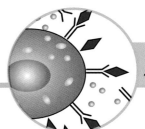

Chapter 11

Anaphylaxis

Introduction

Allergic reactions can be mild to life threatening. Anaphylaxis, by definition, is a sudden, severe, potentially fatal, systemic allergic reaction that can involve various areas of the body (such as the skin, respiratory tract, GI tract, and cardiovascular system). Symptoms occur within minutes to up to 2 hours after contact with the allergy-causing substance but, in rare instances, onset can be delayed for up to 4 hours. Anaphylactoid reactions represent the same process, but are triggered directly without the involvement of IgE molecules. The overall prevalence is 30/100,000 person years. The mortality rate is around 1%. Offending agents include foods, drugs, insect stings, and exercise, but in 20% of the cases, no cause can be found (idiopathic) (*Table 11.1*).

Pathogenesis

Anaphylaxis occurs as a result of degranulation of tissue mast cells and circulating basophils by both IgE-mediated and non-IgE-mediated immunological mechanisms (**11.1**). The resultant release in mediators accounts for the pathophysiological responses seen during anaphylactic reaction (**11.2**).

Table 11.1 Pathogenetic mechanisms and aetiology of anaphylaxis

I IgE-mediated anaphylaxis (60%)
- Drugs: penicillins, cephalosporins, sulphonamides, tetracyclines, quinolones
- Foreign proteins: horse serum, egg albumin, insect venom, enzymes like papain, chymopapain, latex
- Food (30%): eggs, milk, wheat, soy, peanuts, tree nuts, shellfish, apple, peach
- Therapeutic and diagnostic agents: anaesthetic agents, muscle relaxants, hormones
- Allergen immunotherapy
- Exercise-induced anaphylaxis

II Immune complex-mediated anaphylaxis
- Blood and blood products
- Dialysis membranes

III Direct mast cell degranulation
- Opiates, quinolones, vancomycin, muscle relaxants
- Radio contrast media

IV Modulators of arachidonic acid metabolism
- Aspirin, indomethacin

V Idiopathic anaphylaxis
- Exercise
- Catamenial anaphylaxis
- Idiopathic anaphylaxis

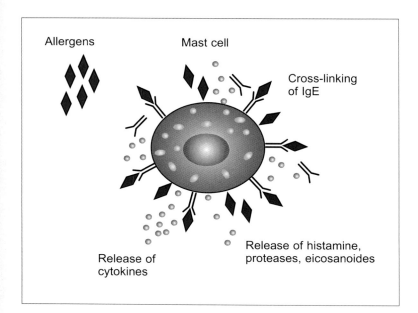

11.1 When mast cells and basophils degranulate, whether by IgE- or non-IgE-mediated mechanisms, pre-formed histamine, and newly generated leukotrienes and prostaglandins are released. The nearly simultaneous explosive release and synthesis of mediators from a large number of cells initiates systemic pathophysiological events, leading to the signs and symptoms of anaphylaxis.

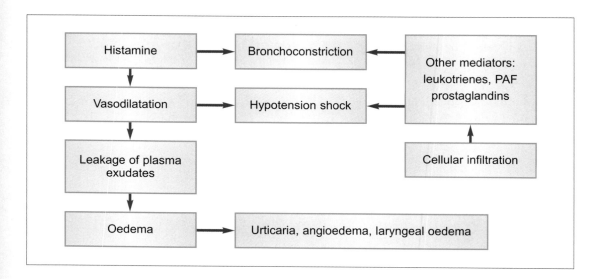

11.2 The pathophysiological responses include smooth muscle spasm in the bronchi and GI tract, vasodilation, increased vascular permeability, and stimulation of sensory nerve endings. These physiological events lead to the classic symptoms of anaphylaxis. (PAF, platelet activating factor.)

Clinical features

Anaphylaxis involves a number of organs and systems. The most common symptoms experienced by patients are cutaneous signs and symptoms, followed by respiratory signs and symptoms in nearly 60% of the affected (*Table 11.2*). Cardiovascular signs and symptoms occur in 33% of the patients. The clinical manifestations in an episode vary widely and may depend on the subject's sensitivity, as well as the amount and type of allergen encountered (**11.3**). The initial symptoms of numbness and tingling of the lips and itching can progress rapidly to generalized urticaria and

angioedema and cardiorespiratory collapse. Death may occur within minutes, and it is usually caused by laryngeal oedema causing stridor, or severe hypotension. Anaphylactic reactions can be confused with other causes of acute onset of generalized urticaria or cardiorespiratory collapse (*Table 11.3*). If there is any doubt regarding the diagnosis, blood should be taken for plasma histamine or serum tryptase levels. Elevated levels indicate mast cell degranulation, and confirm the diagnosis.

Table 11.2 Symptoms and signs of anaphylaxis

- Sense of cutaneous and internal warmth
- Tingling
- Flushing
- Urticaria/angioedema
- Metallic taste in mouth
- Periorbital oedema, erythema
- Wheeze/cough/hoarseness
- Respiratory obstruction and dyspnoea
- Difficulty in swallowing
- Sweating
- Syncope
- Collapse
- Abdominal pain
- Nausea/vomiting/diarrhoea
- Incontinence

Table 11.3 Differential diagnosis of anaphylaxis

- Myocardial infarction
- Pulmonary embolus
- Cardiac arrhythmia
- Vasovagal reaction
- Carcinoid syndrome
- Mastocytosis
- C1 esterase inhibitor deficiency
- Seizure disorder
- Factitious anaphylaxis

The situation most commonly confused with anaphylaxis is vasovagal syncope. As vasovagal syncope can be due to parenteral injections, the confusion with anaphylaxis is more significant. The absence of flushing, pruritus, urticaria, and respiratory difficulties in the presence of bradycardia, and well-preserved blood pressure helps in making the differentiation

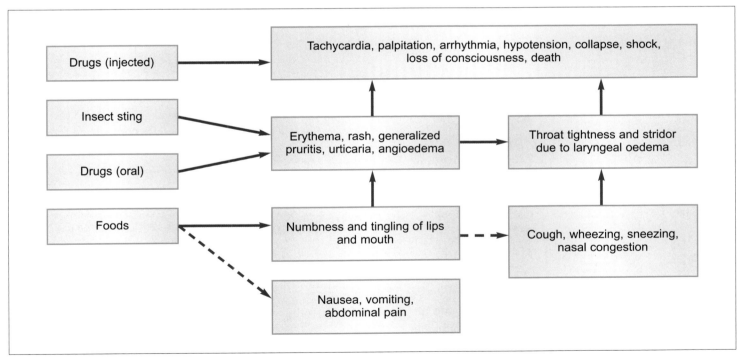

11.3 Clinical presentation of anaphylaxis.

Management

Emergency management of anaphylaxis relies on quick assessment and early treatment. Cardiorespiratory status should be assessed, as in any medical emergency, and appropriate actions should be taken. Once the diagnosis of anaphylaxis is made, epinephrine should be injected intramuscularly into the thigh, as this provides the most efficient absorption. If there is no response to several doses of intramuscular epinephrine, intravenous administration should be considered. Intravenous antihistamine and corticosteroids are given simultaneously (11.4). Drugs commonly used during anaphylaxis are outlined in *Table 11.4*. A short course of corticosteroids is often prescribed to reduce the risk of late-phase reaction, but evidence supporting this is insufficient.

In most cases there is complete resolution of the reaction. However, continued monitoring is essential. If problems persist, further action is required depending on the clinical condition (11.5). Patients receiving certain drugs, such as beta blockers and angiotensin-converting enzyme inhibitors, are at increased risk of inadequate response to the standard treatment.

Patients who have had an anaphylactic reaction should be reviewed in the allergy clinic. If the cause was known, further education and advice on avoidance might be required. If the cause was not known, a detailed history and appropriate investigations reveal the cause in most cases. SPTs or determination of specific IgE helps to confirm the allergen suspected from the history. These include foods, insect stings, and some cases of drug allergies. A challenge may be required in some cases, but this should be done only by physicians experienced in these procedures.

Table 11.4 Drugs used in anaphylaxis

Class of drugs	Agents
Adrenergic stimulants	Epinephrine
	Isoprenaline
	Norepinephrine
	β_2 agonists (nebulized)
	Dopamine
Antihistamines	H1 receptor blockers
	H2 receptor blockers
Xanthines	Aminophylline
Corticosteroids	Hydrocortisone
	Prednisolone

11.4 Patients with known anaphylaxis must carry preloaded devices for administration of epinephrine at all times. Patient education as to the use of a particular device is important. Patients requiring the use of an Epipen should be advised to seek immediate medical help for further management of their anaphylactic event, as additional treatment may be required. Epipen is available in two different strengths: 0.3 ml of 1:1000 solution (for adults), and 0.3 ml of 1:2000 solution (for children).

Recognize
Generalized itching, urticaria, angioedema, stridor, bronchospasm, tachycardia, hypotension, collapse

↓

Immediately
- Lower head, loosen clothing
- Record pulse, blood pressure, respiratory rate
- Establish venous access

↓

Give
- Adrenaline: 500 μg (0.5 ml of 1:1000 solution i.m. (children: 10 μg/kg); repeat every 10 minutes until improvement
- Also give chlorpheniramine 10 mg i.v. and hydrocortisone 200 mg i.v.
- Administer oxygen at 60–100%
- If no improvement; or condition deteriorates, administer adrenaline (1:10,000) 5 ml i.v. (over approx. 5 minutes) under cardiac monitoring. Alternatively, continuous infusion using 1 ml of 1:1000 diluted in 500 ml of 5% dextrose infused at a rate of 0.25–2.5 ml/min

Continue to monitor O_2 saturation, pulse and blood pressure

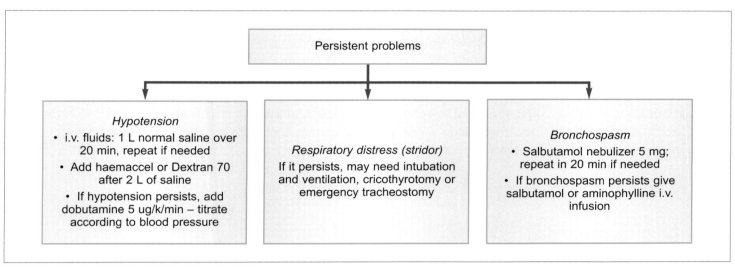

11.5 Subsequent management of anaphylaxis.

Prevention

The dramatic and potentially fatal nature of anaphylaxis makes its prevention the primary clinical goal. Patients who have anaphylaxis should have their specific cause identified. Total abstinence from the inciting allergen is the best way to eliminate the risk of anaphylaxis. Patients with anaphylaxis should receive written instructions on allergen avoidance and cross-sensitive materials. Education must extend to lifestyles and activity modification. Patients who have experienced anaphylaxis should be discouraged from using angiotensin-converting enzyme inhibitors and beta blockers. Patients with exercise-induced anaphylaxis should be advised to exercise only in the morning after an overnight fast, as many of these patients require the ingestion of any food, or sometimes a specific food, prior to experiencing anaphylaxis.

Those who are at continued risk of inadvertent exposures (e.g. to foods, such as nuts), should carry self-injectable epinephrine and antihistamines, and be educated in its use (**11.6**). If exposure can not be avoided (e.g. to certain drugs,

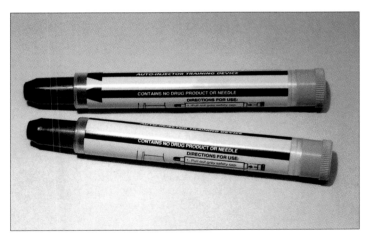

11.6 Epipen for the emergency administration of epinephrine and antihistamine.

such as penicillin or insulin), desensitization can be attempted (*Table 11.5*). Desensitization involves administration of a known allergen or drug in incremental doses. Desensitization has to be carried out in a controlled environment, as systemic and even fatal reactions can occur. Allergen immunotherapy has been evaluated in various studies, and has been found to be particularly useful in Hymenoptera sensitivity. Immunotherapy has not proven to

be useful in the treatment of food allergy or antibiotic-mediated anaphylaxis.

Pre-medication prior to interaction with a known inciting agent is useful in managing patients with sensitivity to radio contrast media. Patients suffering from idiopathic anaphylaxis are best managed with regular oral sympathomimetics, antihistaminics, and glucocorticoids.

Table 11.5 Methods for prevention of anaphylaxis

- Allergen avoidance
- Patient education
- Epipen
- Desensitization
- Beta stimulants
- Allergen immunotherapy
- Pre-medication with glucocorticoids and antihistamines
- Regular oral sympathomimetics, glucocorticoids, antihistaminics in idiopathic anaphylaxis
- DNA vaccines

Index